Mary Burgess has worked as a cognitive behavioural therapist with patients with severe fatigue including chronic fatigue syndrome (CFS) for more than twenty years. In addition to her clinical work she has been engaged in research and development. This involved developing and evaluating interventions for adults and adolescents who experienced difficulty in getting to the hospital due to the severity of their symptoms. With colleagues, this work has been published in academic journals and led to the writing of the original version of this book.

Trudie Chalder is Professor of Cognitive Behavioural Psychotherapy at King's College London. She has worked as a clinician and a researcher in the area of fatigue for about thirty years. She developed the cognitive behavioural treatment of CFS and the approach has now been evaluated in a number of clinical research trials with positive results.

D0933104

The aim of the **Overcoming** series is to enable people with a range of common problems and disorders to take control of their own recovery programme.

Each title, with its specially tailored programme, is devised by a practising clinician using the latest techniques of cognitive behavioural therapy – techniques that have been shown to be highly effective in changing the way patients think about themselves and their problems.

Many books in the **Overcoming** series are recommended under the Reading Well scheme.

Other titles in the series include:

OVERCOMING ALCOHOL MISUSE, 2ND EDITION
OVERCOMING ANGER AND IRRITABILITY, 2ND EDITION
OVERCOMING ANOREXIA NERVOSA
OVERCOMING ANXIETY, 2ND EDITION
OVERCOMING BODY IMAGE PROBLEMS INCLUDING
DYSMORPHIC DISORDER
OVERCOMING BULIMIA NERVOSA AND BINGE-EATING, 3RD EDITION
OVERCOMING CHILDHOOD TRAUMA
OVERCOMING CHRONIC PAIN
OVERCOMING DEPERSONALISATION AND FEELINGS OF
UNREALITY, 2ND EDITION
OVERCOMING GAMBLING ADDICTION, 2ND EDITION
OVERCOMING GRIEF
OVERCOMING HEALTH ANXIETY
OVERCOMING HOARDING
OVERCOMING INSOMNIA AND SLEEP PROBLEMS
OVERCOMING LOW SELF-ESTEEM, 2ND EDITION
OVERCOMING MILD TRAUMATIC BRAIN INJURY AND
POST-CONCUSSION SYMPTOMS
OVERCOMING MOOD SWINGS
OVERCOMING OBSESSIVE COMPULSIVE DISORDER
OVERCOMING PANIC, 2ND EDITION
OVERCOMING PARANOID AND
SUSPICIOUS THOUGHTS, 2ND EDITION
OVERCOMING PERFECTIONISM, 2ND EDITION
OVERCOMING RELATIONSHIP PROBLEMS, 2ND EDITION
OVERCOMING SEXUAL PROBLEMS, 2ND EDITION
OVERCOMING SOCIAL ANXIETY AND SHYNESS, 2ND EDITION
OVERCOMING STRESS
OVERCOMING TRAUMATIC STRESS, 2ND EDITION
OVERCOMING WEIGHT PROBLEMS
OVERCOMING WORRY AND GENERALISED ANXIETY DISORDER,
2ND EDITION
OVERCOMING YOUR CHILD'S FEARS AND WORRIES
OVERCOMING YOUR CHILD'S SHYNESS AND SOCIAL ANXIETY
STOP SMOKING NOW, 2ND EDITION

OVERCOMING CHRONIC FATIGUE

2nd Edition

A self-help guide using
cognitive behavioural techniques

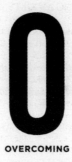

OVERCOMING

MARY BURGESS

with

TRUDIE CHALDER

ROBINSON

ROBINSON

First published in Great Britain in 2005 by Robinson, an imprint of
Constable & Robinson Ltd

This revised and updated edition published in 2019 by Robinson

A CIP catalogue record for this book
is available from the British Library.

Important Note
This book is not intended as a substitute for medical advice or treatment.
Any person with a condition requiring medical attention should consult a
qualified medical practitioner or suitable therapist.

ISBN: 978-1-47213-885-9

Typeset in Bembo by Initial Typesetting Services, Edinburgh
Printed and bound in Great Britain by CPI Group (UK), Croydon CR0 4YY

Papers used by Robinson are from well-managed forests and
other responsible sources

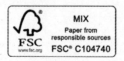

Robinson
An imprint of
Little, Brown Book Group
Carmelite House
50 Victoria Embankment
London EC4Y 0DZ

An Hachette UK Company
www.hachette.co.uk
www.littlebrown.co.uk

Contents

PART THREE:
Making Further Progress

PART FOUR:
How Others Can Help

Acknowledgements

This second edition of *Overcoming Chronic Fatigue* has been developed over the course of many years and a huge number of people have contributed to the final product. We would like first to mention those many people with chronic fatigue who have used the techniques described in the first edition and have made suggestions on how our book could be improved. We would also like to thank our colleagues, past and present, who have commented on the text.

The source of the physiological explanation of chronic fatigue syndrome and some of the information contained within the section on autonomic arousal in CFS came from an unpublished treatment manual written by Pauline Powell, a physiotherapist in Liverpool.

The chapter on overcoming unhelpful thinking patterns was originally influenced by work carried out by Christine Padesky and Dennis Greenberger; for more comprehensive explanations of the ideas contained within this chapter, we recommend that you refer to their book *Mind over Mood* (for details see Chapter 14, 'Useful resources'). Iram Sattar, a GP who has a special interest in different cultural needs, contributed to the section on cultural issues.

Abigale Childs, an MSC student, assisted us with the chapter on 'Useful resources'.

Foreword

by one of Mary's former clients

The tools, exercises and guidance in this book <u>work</u>.

So much so that they saved my life.

That may seem a grand and incredible statement, but I can honestly say it's true.

I had tried several other reputable 'avenues' to help me with the fatigue and challenges I was experiencing, but the unfortunate truth is they did not work and actually made things considerably worse.

Enter CBT and Dr Mary Burgess.

This book is, as described, the self-help version of the CBT programme I had the great fortune of participating in directly with Mary.

Mary never went by her formal title, Dr Burgess, and she is not like any other doctor or health practitioner I've ever come across.

She never used a 'doctor-knows-all' approach. Instead, she worked *with* me in the way *I* needed to be able to move forward, make progress and, ultimately and most importantly, recover.

To give you a better picture of Mary, she would show up to my house for a session – I was housebound at the time – in her cycling gear, having cycled from the CFS Unit at King's College Hospital here in London.

No white coat.

Instead, black cycle shorts, cycling shoes complete with toe clips, a colorful cycle top, her helmet and some yellow-tinted shades (so she could see the road better).

No authoritarian attitude.

Instead, a genuinely caring demeanour, a constructive and gently challenging approach, a hopeful and optimistic out-look and, ultimately, a deep and steadfast belief that I *could and would get better*, even at those times when I had lost all hope myself and **could** not even remotely see that I could ever be well again.

And here I am.

Writing this.

For you.

As the proof in the pudding.

You may not have the great fortune of working directly with Mary, but this book is her life's work, all twenty-four years of it, condensed into this beautifully simple and incredibly powerful programme to help you get better and be well.

I truly hope that you are not as unwell as I was (housebound with a wide range of symptoms), but if you are, you can rest assured that the programme outlined in this book will help you to be well again.

It was hard, I won't lie, but I look back now at the challenging things I had to wade through and the small steps I had to take that seemed utterly impossible and honestly? I smile.

To give you a concrete example, at one point after having been so housebound, I was petrified about going outside again. I had completely lost my self-confidence in being able to do things. Walking to my front gate, which was a mere fourteen steps from my front door, felt totally overwhelming and seemed altogether impossible.

AND YET!

Through the use of the tools, especially focusing on one of my targets (short walks) and using the unhelpful patterns of thinking descriptions (especially the catastrophising one), I was able to make it to the front gate and back.

What a huge accomplishment that was!

As I look back on that day now, yes, walking to the gate seemed an incredibly small step, and yet, in reality, it was huge.

And that's the key to this book.

Small steps, seemingly infinitesimal steps – literally and metaphorically – are how you will get better.

(After walking to the gate, my next step became the nearest tree just beyond the front gate. And then the next tree and the next tree, all the way up to now when I am walking a good two to three miles easily and playing football with my son in the park.)

Equally, small, seemingly infinitesimal changes in your beliefs are how you will shift the underlying foundation of who you are.

The downward arrow technique really works!

At first I couldn't even remotely believe the new core beliefs I had replaced the old ones with.

Now I do.

And you can too!

The pie chart exercise or 'life pie' as I like to call it?

It's a wonderful companion to my new core beliefs and a great way to help me keep my perspective on the various aspects of my life and, most importantly, maintain balance so that I don't 'crash and burn' any more.

I honestly would never want to go back to where I was.

But I know now that the doubt and fear that I could never get better was totally unfounded.

Why?

Again, because here I am.

So let this book be your Mary.

Let it guide you and help you.

Let it be the one 'thing' that helps you get better and be well.

And, if I may be so bold as to offer some of my own wisdom

alongside the pearls and practicality in these pages, it would be this:

1) Your body is your best friend

It never has and never will betray you. It's always on your side, always there for you. Your body can't speak in words, so it uses symptoms as messages. Fatigue or tiredness is simply your body trying to tell you to change something, to honour yourself more, to be kinder to yourself. I constantly berated myself for feeling so tired and being so housebound. Now I realise that that was only compounding things, so instead of being my own worst enemy, I'm now my own best friend. BFF are we!

2) I can't do that <u>YET</u>

When your self-confidence wanes and the target you have in mind seems like the highest of mountains you'll never reach, let YET be your go-to hiking buddy. 'I can't do that' becomes 'I can't do that YET'. Feel the difference? Without YET, we're looking at an impossible peak, a closed door: no hope, no possibility, certain failure. With our friend YET, the door may be only slightly ajar, but oh my, there's a beautiful sliver of light shining through it and oh, the possibilities! We can reach that peak!

3) It's all in the small

Alongside our favourite hiking buddy YET, chunking things down into the *smallest* possible steps was the 'magic sauce' that helped me make progress. Breaking down your targets into teeny tiny steps really works! By making the step as small as possible, not only did it mean I could *achieve* it, it also helped me to nurture my *self-confidence* and *self-belief* that I could do it. And so I did.

4) Celebrate along the way!

It's good to keep your target or goal in mind, but don't let the end undermine the means. If you take what might seem like an infinitesimal, insignificant step, celebrate it! Clichéd as it may sound, give yourself a pat on the back or a hug or whatever kind of recognition and kindness towards yourself that is validating and celebratory. You deserve it and yes, you're worth it!

5) If you don't like the layout, lay it out differently

At first, I could not fill out the sleep and activity diaries at all. It was as if they were staring at me, cold and blank and menacing. When I did have a go at filling them out, which was excruciating, they glared at me even harder, only this time with what I perceived as failure after failure. The solution to that for me? Lay it out differently! I'm an inherently creative, design-conscious and picture-brained person, so completing the diaries with coloured pens and using sticky notes made the world of difference for me. Suddenly the diaries were my friends, encouraging me and cheering me on!

6) Love yourself like nobody's business

Because, really, it isn't anyone else's business and it's the most important 'business' you'll ever have. As I slowly disrupted and let go of the constant stream of negative self-talk and unhelpful thinking patterns, I started instead to give myself compassion and love. Even today, instead of going into a hypercritical tirade when I make a mistake, I remind myself that everyone makes mistakes and really, it's OK. And it is.

7) Let in the good

If there are moments or days or even weeks when you're feeling so awful you can't do very much at all, focus your attention on a few small *good* things. Even just one is enough. For me that was sunshine streaming through the window, hearing a bird sing, the tree across from our house, petting our dog, enjoying the scent of an essential oil, reading a few pages in a book, gazing at the stars. Whatever the good might be for you, let it in. And *let it linger*. It will remind you of who you are and how you can be.

8) You are not alone

One of the hardest aspects of experiencing such debilitating fatigue was the isolation. Being housebound obviously meant no going out, no seeing friends, nothing. This made me feel even worse about myself and it also meant my negative automatic thoughts ran rampant. (Unhelpful thinking patterns exercises to the rescue!) One of the most helpful antidotes to this feeling of isolation was hearing about other individuals who had experienced fatigue and how they navigated this very hard terrain. It made me feel less alone and it also made me realise that what I was experiencing was actually *normal*. Not that I would wish this kind of fatigue on anyone, but may my and the other stories in this book be an inspiration and solace for you and, most importantly, help you to know that you are most definitely not alone.

9) Believe you can and you will

Believe that you *can* get better and you *will*. For a long time I did not think I could ever get better. I couldn't see any kind of future where I was actually well and could do things again. That was a dark, deep place and it was hard to see any kind of way forward. So if you are there, or even if you are not, please let this book be your beacon. Mary held a torch of hope for me when I could not. You can get better. Step by infinitesimal step. And this book, and Mary through it, will be there with you every step of the way.

Now all of this may seem like an awfully long to-do list. But none of it is intended as anything you have to do as part of the programme described in these pages.

If anything, the above is an invitation for how to be while making your way through the programme outlined in this book.

You are your own point of power.

Always.

Mary can guide you and the information, tools, exercises and guidance in this book can help you recover from the fatigue you are experiencing.

But remember:

You have the power to change your life, to recover, to be truly and vibrantly well.

And with that, dear reader, I'm off to meet a friend for lunch and then pick up my son from school (and walk home together!), things I could barely even dream of a few years ago.

May you be well, and may you too once again enjoy the things that make your heart sing.

Preface

Fatigue is central to many chronic and debilitating illnesses, including chronic fatigue syndrome, chronic pain, cancer, inflammatory diseases and chronic respiratory problems. However, fatigue can also occur when we are overcommitted, working too hard or not sleeping well.

We are delighted to have been given the opportunity to write a second edition of this book. Our reasons for writing the original self-help book were varied. First, we had carried out a small research study at King's College Hospital, London, which indicated that some patients improved after using a version of this self-help book with only phone calls from a therapist. Second, there are people who do not have access to a clinician with the expertise to help them to overcome their fatigue-related problems. Finally, some people have difficulty attending regular appointments. This may be due to the severity of their symptoms, distance or time restrictions due to work or family commitments. Changes that we have made to this second edition have come about following further research, feedback from clinicians and, most importantly, people who have used this book either alone or with a therapist. Note that names have occasionally been changed in the text to ensure anonymity.

You may notice as you read through this book that we make a number of references to chronic fatigue syndrome and indeed have included a chapter on it. We have done this because originally that was the main reason for referral to the unit. However, over the past ten years or so, people have been coming to see us for fatigue due to other reasons as well and we have been helping them with strategies outlined in this book.

The overall aim of this book is to help you to overcome your fatigue and other related symptoms and improve the quality of your life.

The advice provided in this book may be enough to help some people feel better; however, it may not be sufficient for everyone. Advice on where to get further help is offered in Chapter 14 on 'Useful resources'.

How to use this book

The information in this book has been laid out in an order that people generally find useful. We therefore recommend that you work your way through the book in the order that it has been written. We have suggested a programme of steps to guide you on your journey. Please see the table on pages 108–9. However, if you come to a chapter that you do not feel is relevant, do leave it out. You can always come back to it.

In most of the chapters, we ask you to keep some diaries; you may photocopy the blanks provided for your own use. However, if you do not like the format of the diaries, you are welcome to devise something similar that works better for you.

If you know someone who is keen to support you, Chapter 15, 'Some guidelines for partners, relatives and friends', may be helpful.

What does this book include?

This book is divided into four parts:

Part One aims to help you to understand more about your own fatigue problem. It describes factors that many people with chronic fatigue syndrome report around the time that their fatigue began, and then discusses factors that commonly appear to be involved in maintaining it.

Part Two is divided into ten chapters that describe a variety of practical strategies that aim to help you overcome your fatigue problems. We ask you to consider 'A few words of warning!' on page 49, just to be sure that this approach is right for you.

Part Three focuses on helping you to consolidate what you have learned and suggests ways to help you to maintain and build on your progress.

Information on where to get further help and a reading list are also provided.

Finally, Part Four offers some brief guidelines and information for people close to you such as your partner, relatives and close friends. The aim of this chapter is to help those people to understand your fatigue problems and to offer you support as and when you need it.

PART ONE

UNDERSTANDING CHRONIC FATIGUE SYNDROME

1

What is chronic fatigue syndrome?

In this chapter, we give you some background information about chronic fatigue syndrome and discuss factors that may contribute to its onset. We also offer some explanations for many of the common symptoms experienced by people with chronic fatigue syndrome and discuss some of the treatments that are available.

What is fatigue?

Fatigue is a difficult concept as it means different things to different people. People will often describe their fatigue using words such as *weakness*, *listlessness*, *profound tiredness* or *sleepiness*, a *complete lack of energy* or *feeling totally drained*. Fatigue feels very different from the normal sort of tiredness experienced by a healthy person.

Fatigue is a very common problem. It is a symptom that can be associated with many illnesses, including chronic pain, thyroid problems, anaemia and cancer. A single explanation for fatigue is rarely found but sometimes develops following a viral infection such as glandular fever and sometimes occurs when life is very busy and stressful. Whatever the cause of fatigue, it is a *real* and debilitating problem.

What is chronic fatigue syndrome?

Chronic fatigue syndrome (CFS), also known as post-viral fatigue syndrome (PVFS) or myalgic encephalomyelitis (ME), is an illness that has attracted much attention over recent years. Agreeing a name for the illness has been problematic as there has been much debate about the relative contributions of 'physiological' and 'psychological' factors in its development. This outmoded, dualistic view of illness assumes that the body and mind work separately and is unhelpful in understanding any condition. We will be offering alternative ways of viewing CFS later on.

Chronic fatigue syndrome is a relatively new label, although the illness itself was clearly described more than a hundred years ago; at that time, it was called *neurasthenia*.

The main symptom experienced by people with CFS is persistent mental and physical fatigue that feels overwhelming and unlike normal tiredness. Other symptoms may include painful muscles and/or joints, sore throat, headaches, pins and needles, dizziness and sensitivity to light and noise. CFS has some marked similarities to fibromyalgia, a disorder involving widespread musculoskeletal pain and fatigue; however, the component of muscle pain in fibromyalgia is generally higher.

People with CFS often report impairments of their

4

thinking, such as poor concentration, difficulty in finding words and impaired short-term memory. People will sometimes describe feeling 'woolly-headed'. Problems with sleep are also common: for example, difficulty getting to sleep, sleeping for very long periods, restless sleep with frequent dreams, waking frequently and waking feeling unrefreshed. Many people with CFS also report digestive disturbances such as bloating, nausea or loss of appetite. Food intolerances and increased sensitivity to some foods, alcohol and substances containing caffeine, such as tea and coffee, are often reported.

Symptoms vary among individuals and affect their lives in different ways. For some people this may mean giving up work or studying; alternatively, or in addition, it may mean reducing or restricting social and/or leisure activities. Life at home can change: for example, you may be able to do less chores or cooking or be less able to help care for children. Personal relationships may change, with less inclination or energy for intimacy. The severity of symptoms may lead a small percentage of people with CFS to be housebound for much of the time. Symptoms are often made worse by physical and mental exertion and sometimes by stress. The impact of symptoms may for some people lead them to feel anxious and/or low in mood.

How is chronic fatigue syndrome diagnosed?

As with many other illnesses where there is no known single cause – for example, irritable bowel syndrome (IBS) – there is no test to diagnose chronic fatigue syndrome. A diagnosis of CFS is usually made by taking a detailed account of the symptoms, including how they started, how they behave (e.g. whether they worsen in response to certain activities) and the length of time they have been occurring. Basic screening blood tests will also be carried out to rule out any other illnesses that may account for the symptoms. Other more specialist tests are sometimes conducted – for example, if there has been a recent significant weight loss or a history of foreign travel prior to the onset of symptoms. Medical practitioners can make the diagnosis of CFS, but sometimes they prefer to refer patients to a specialist with an interest in CFS.

How common is chronic fatigue syndrome?

It is difficult to say precisely how common chronic fatigue syndrome is in the general population. First, it depends on how chronic fatigue syndrome is defined. Second, although some people may have all the symptoms of CFS, they may not attribute them to the illness itself.

Although 10–30 per cent of all UK patients going to see their doctor for any reason report substantial fatigue lasting for more than a few weeks (15–27 per cent in the US), studies have indicated that a diagnosis of chronic fatigue syndrome is made in only a small minority of these cases. CFS appears to be more common in women than men. A variety of explanations have been put forward for this, in particular changes in the role of women, with increased demands and expectations. Although fatigue is relatively uncommon during childhood, its incidence rises during adolescence.

Chronic fatigue syndrome can occur at any time in adulthood.

What causes chronic fatigue syndrome?

As we noted above, there is no single cause of CFS. People report a variety of different things that happened at the beginning of their illness. Some people can pinpoint the exact date that their CFS started; for others, the onset is more gradual. In light of this wide range of experience, it is unlikely that a single cause for CFS will ever be identified. However, there is a growing body of evidence suggesting that a number of factors may be involved in triggering the illness.

If you have chronic fatigue syndrome, it is likely that you will be able to identify some, though probably not all, of the triggers listed below. There may be factors that we have not included that you feel are relevant to the onset of your fatigue.

Infection

The starting point of CFS is often associated with an initial illness, frequently in the form of a viral infection: for example, glandular fever. Serious viral infections such as glandular fever can make us feel tired for up to six months.

Sometimes people report having had a series of infections, which may be a sign that they are run down. However,

7

there is no clear evidence of the virus or bacterium persisting once CFS has become established. Recent research suggests that excessive resting at the height of an infection is likely to lead to worse symptoms several weeks and months later. Although it is advisable to 'take it easy' when in the acute phase of an infection, too much rest is unhelpful.

Lifestyle

Fatigue can develop in association with a busy lifestyle. Leading a life that allows little opportunity for relaxation is stressful, even though at the time it may feel manageable and possibly exhilarating. Following an infection or other illness, a person may feel under pressure to meet their previous levels of commitment, whether at work or at home, and this may lead to exhaustion. Being too busy is as likely to lead to fatigue as being inactive.

Life events

Changing jobs, getting married, moving house, leaving home (e.g. to begin university), a bereavement, ending a long-term relationship: all these are stressful events that may lead to increased vulnerability to CFS.

Personality

People with CFS often report that they are hardworking and conscientious, and have high expectations of themselves.

Individuals with this type of personality tend to strive very hard to achieve in all they do, leaving little time for pleasure or relaxation.

What keeps the chronic fatigue problem going?

Just as there are a number of factors involved in triggering CFS, there are also likely to be many factors involved in keeping it going. Your own story is unique, but you may feel that some of the following factors may apply to your situation.

Resuming normal activities too soon after an initial infection

If you keep up your usual level of activity when you have an infection or another illness, or resume that level almost immediately, then your recovery is likely to take longer as your body is working extra hard.

Resting too much

Although resting for a short time is the correct thing to do when you have an acute illness or infection, prolonged rest can impede recovery and cause its own set of problems. Evidence suggests that the longer you rest when you have a viral illness, the more symptoms you will have six months later. Prolonged rest makes it harder to become active again and actually increases fatigue. Resting for too long will affect the cardiovascular system, nervous system and musculoskeletal system. Further details of the physical effects of CFS are given on pages 13–25 in the section titled 'Physiological aspects of chronic fatigue syndrome'.

Receiving confusing messages about the illness itself and how to deal with it

Many people with CFS will have sought advice or treatment from a variety of sources. They may have been given different messages, which can be confusing. People report often being told by well-meaning health professionals that they should rest at the onset and have frequently been encouraged to rest for too long. This advice is often accompanied by fear-inducing messages that not resting will lead to prolonged illness. This can all too easily leave the person feeling baffled about what to do for the best and further wearied by the effort of trying to find a potential 'cure'.

Over-vigorous activity alternating with resting for long periods

Some people refer to this as a 'boom and bust pattern', by which we mean, doing too much when you have some energy, resulting in feeling more fatigued and having to rest for longer afterwards. This pattern of activity exacerbates the problem in the longer term, as it makes it difficult to establish any type of routine.

Disturbed sleep pattern

A disturbed or erratic sleep pattern is very common in people with CFS and undoubtedly this increases feelings of fatigue and other related symptoms. Factors that may contribute to a disturbed sleep pattern include going to bed and/or getting up at irregular times, resting or sleeping for long periods in the day worrying, or having an active mind at bedtime.

Focusing on symptoms

The symptoms commonly experienced by people with CFS are both distressing and debilitating, and it is therefore understandable that from time to time you may worry about them. Unfortunately, symptoms thrive on attention: in other words, the more you focus on them, the worse they are likely to feel.

Worries about activity making your symptoms worse

People with CFS commonly experience increased fatigue or pain after *any* activity, and many understandably read this as a sign that they are doing harm to their bodies. If you have worries like these, you may have understandably reduced your activities and be resting for long periods in the belief that resting will help you to feel better. However, as we have already mentioned, resting for too long can cause its own set of problems.

Life stress and low mood

Many people with CFS experience significant and continuing stresses and problems in their lives due to the impact of their symptoms. These may include one or more of the following:

- financial difficulties arising from having given up work or reduced working hours;
- worries about holding down a job or keeping up with studies;
- anxiety about a changed role within the family through being less able to take responsibility for dependants;
- reduced social contacts, leading to feelings of isolation;
- feelings of guilt about not being a 'good' parent because of being unable to do the things you used to do, e.g., playing, helping with homework, going out for the day, etc.;
- relationship issues such as feeling uneasy or guilty that your partner has to do more than previously to help you out or that you are unable to be as spontaneous or go out as much.

These stresses and anxieties can understandably trigger feelings such as frustration, helplessness and a sense of loss of control over life. Sometimes these feelings can lead to low mood, and even to depression. Low mood can further exacerbate fatigue and lead to reduced motivation and also a difficulty in enjoying things.

Physiological aspects of chronic fatigue syndrome

Many people with CFS are concerned that their distressing symptoms may be related to a disease that hasn't been detected. Others, who had a viral infection at the time their CFS began, are sometimes concerned that the virus is still present or has caused damage to the body. Intensive research has tried to establish a physiological explanation for the very distressing and debilitating symptoms experienced by people with CFS.

Over time, reduced or irregular activity and increased periods of rest cause physical changes in the body. These changes can both exacerbate the unpleasant sensations of CFS and cause additional symptoms such as increased muscle pain during exercise. It is important to point out that these changes are reversible with physical rehabilitation and/or exercise.

Researchers have looked at the effects of rest on healthy people when they reduce their activities, and many similarities between healthy inactive people and people with CFS have been noted. The following paragraphs describe the effects of prolonged periods of inactivity on the body, and how these effects are experienced.

Changes in muscle function

A decrease in the number of active cell mitochondria (tiny parts of the cell that produce energy) and their enzymes has been found in the muscles of CFS patients when compared with healthy *active* people. This reduction of cell mitochondria has also been found in healthy *inactive* people. Fewer cell mitochondria may lead to production of lactic acid at low levels of exercise, which in turn limits muscle performance.

These changes may account for the feeling of a lack of power or energy in the muscles.

Reduced activity leads to muscles being less efficient (reduced in strength, tone and size), and consequently less effective in squeezing the blood back to the heart; this causes blood to pool in the lower part of the legs.

Pooling of blood can cause pain both during activity and at rest.

When muscles are not used regularly, they become unfit or deconditioned. When these muscles contract during activity, uneven stresses are produced.

This may result in a feeling of weakness and unsteadiness followed by delayed pain and discomfort.

In respect of this last point, it is important to note that, for everyone, muscle pain and stiffness are natural consequences of beginning a new exercise programme or taking exercise to which they are unaccustomed. They are therefore not an indication that the exercise should be halted; only that it should be carried out consistently and built up gradually.

Changes in the cardiovascular system

The cardiovascular system (which incorporates the heart and blood vessels) loses condition very quickly with rest. The longer you rest, the more changes occur.

Physical changes that occur with cardiovascular deconditioning include:

- after one or two days' bed rest, reduced blood volume;
- after eight days' bed rest, reduced volume of red blood cells, which reduces the oxygen-carrying capacity of the blood;
- after twenty days' bed rest, the volume of the heart reduces by about 15 per cent, so that less blood is pumped to other organs.

The physical changes described above may result in making you feel breathless or dizzy when exercising, and contribute to your fatigue.

Following a 'lying down' rest, there is a drop in blood pressure on standing up (postural hypotension) as gravity causes blood to pool in the limbs. Consequently, less blood returns to the heart and therefore less blood goes to the brain. Restricting salt or liquid intake reduces blood volume and can exacerbate dizziness on standing up.

The reduced blood flow to the brain causes dizziness and sometimes fainting on standing up.

Regulation of body temperature

Changes in the blood flow to major body organs occur following prolonged rest, and these lead to changes in surface body temperature.

This may result in feeling hot and/or cold, with excessive and inappropriate sweating at times.

Changes in sight and hearing

Prolonged bed rest results in a 'headward' shift of bodily fluids.

This may result in visual problems and sensitivity to noise.

Reduced tolerance to activity or exercise

General deconditioning of the body occurs as a result of prolonged rest or reduced activity.

As fitness reduces, it is harder work to be active. Muscle fatigue and feelings of heaviness, as well as a general increase in overall fatigue, occur when activity is resumed.

During periods of prolonged physical or mental exertion, the nervous system is more active than normal and adrenaline production is raised. This leads to symptoms similar to those experienced in a flu-like illness, such as *aches and pains, headache, sweating, feeling hot and cold, chest tightness* and *sore throat*. If a person experiences these symptoms after activity, they may reduce or avoid activities, as they may believe that they are coming down with flu or a cold. Limiting activity can perpetuate the symptoms and lead to a further reduction of fitness and muscle strength.

Changes in the nervous system

One of the functions of the nervous system is to coordinate the muscles. Regular performance of an activity is required to maintain good coordination. Prolonged periods of inactivity therefore reduce coordination.

This may result in unsteadiness, clumsiness and reduced accuracy on carrying out precise movements.

Changes in mental functioning

Prolonged rest deprives people of intellectual stimulation and has a dulling effect on intellectual activity.

This may impair concentration, memory and the ability to find the correct word.

Alteration of the biological clock

The 'biological clock', which is located in a part of the brain called the hypothalamus, regulates many body rhythms that run on an approximate twenty-four-hour cycle. These rhythms are called 'circadian rhythms', and they control vital functions such as:

- sleeping and waking;
- feelings of tiredness and alertness;
- intellectual performance;
- memory;
- appetite;
- body temperature;
- the production of hormones e.g. cortisol (which is important in regulating our metabolism);
- the activity of the immune system.

Circadian rhythms are responsible for the body 'feeling'

things at certain times of the day: for example, hunger, alertness, tiredness, the need to go to the bathroom. The biological clock is affected by the events of the day and is reset each day by cues such as times of getting up or going to bed, mealtimes and performing daily routines. If these cues do not occur, the biological clock's timekeeping can be disturbed; this can happen, for example, when flying across different time-zones (jet-lag), working shifts – or experiencing illness.

If regular cues are lost, disruption of the clock results in a slipping of body rhythms that can lead to:

- the 'normal' intense feelings of tiredness at night shifting into the day, making it difficult to cope with your usual daytime routine;
- the 'normal' daytime rhythm shifting to the night, making you more alert and causing difficulty in getting to sleep.

This in turn can lead to:

- poor-quality sleep at night;
- increasing fatigue during the day;
- poor concentration and forgetfulness;
- low mood;
- feeling generally unwell;
- headaches;
- muscle aches;
- loss of appetite;
- irregularities of bowel movement.

As the symptoms of chronic fatigue syndrome are similar to those of jet-lag, circadian rhythms of people with CFS have been investigated. Evidence from some studies indicates that CFS is associated with the biological clock losing control of the body rhythms.

What may happen is an infection, a very stressful life event, or an accumulation of persistent stress causes worry and disturbs sleep at night. This leads to irregular times of getting up and going to bed, and more rests taken during the day. Thus, the usual daily routine and normal sleep–waking cycle, both needed to reset the biological clock, are disrupted. The biological clock then loses control over body rhythms, resulting in the mental and physical symptoms of CFS.

Disturbance of cortisol production

Cortisol is a hormone whose production is controlled by a circadian rhythm. It sets our metabolism in action in the morning to prepare us for the physical and mental challenges of the day. Exercise, other activity and stress cause an increase in the level of cortisol in the bloodstream.

Low cortisol levels have been found in people who have disrupted sleep, such as healthy individuals who have rested in bed for more than three weeks, healthy workers after working five-night shifts and people suffering from jet-lag.

Research shows that some people with CFS also have a lower than normal level of cortisol; it is thought that these low cortisol levels are probably associated with disrupted sleep and irregular activity.

Low cortisol may add to the feeling of tiredness, decreased alertness and poor performance seen both in people with CFS and in those who work on night shifts.

Disturbance of the sleep-wake rhythm

Most people with CFS complain of poor-quality sleep. Common problems include difficulty in getting to sleep, restlessness, waking in the night and waking feeling unrefreshed and sleepy.

In a study where the sleep patterns of healthy volunteers were deliberately disrupted to make them similar to those of people with CFS, they developed symptoms similar to those of CFS, including feeling unrefreshed and physically weak, sleepiness, poor concentration and muscle aches.

However, when they were allowed to sleep undisturbed, their symptoms subsided. This study indicates that a disturbed sleep pattern can cause some symptoms of CFS, but that these symptoms are reversible.

Disruption of sleep can affect the activity of the immune system, possibly increasing vulnerability to colds and infection.

Inactivity and being deprived of sleep cause an increase in the feelings of effort and fatigue when performing activity or exercise.

Autonomic arousal in chronic fatigue syndrome

Autonomic arousal is an automatic physical response of

the body to a threatening or stressful situation. We can all remember having butterflies before an exam, an interview, or going to the dentist! When we are in a situation that makes us feel anxious, the central nervous system becomes more active and an increased amount of the hormone adrenaline is released into the bloodstream. These natural changes have a protective function in preparing us for action to counter a threatened danger; however, the physical feelings that we experience when anxious can be very unpleasant.

Having CFS can at times be very stressful. As well as dealing with your illness, you may also be facing other concerns related to it, such as financial worries and/or an inability to meet deadlines at work, college or home. You may worry about whether you are making your symptoms worse by following advice that you have been given. You also may worry about the causes of your condition and the effects of CFS on your own and others' lives. If you have been ill for a long time, you may worry about doing things that you haven't done for a while, such as meeting friends. All of these worries may at times trigger feelings of anxiety, which in turn can lead to a range of unpleasant physical feelings. These effects, and how you may experience them, are listed below.

Increased heart rate

This can be felt as a racing pulse, palpitations, pounding, or tightness in the chest.

Some people feel very frightened by these sensations and so become yet more anxious, resulting in a further release of adrenaline that maintains the physical sensations.

Increase in blood pressure

High blood pressure is noted in some people with anxiety. This is likely to be associated with an exaggerated autonomic response to stress by the nervous system.

There are usually no particular signs or symptoms of high blood pressure; it is usually detected only in the course of routine investigations by doctors or if another illness is present: for example, heart or kidney problems.

Breathlessness, which can lead to hyperventilation

This natural response to being anxious enables our lungs to be filled with oxygen to prepare us for action. However, if over-breathing (hyperventilation) continues for a while, an array of unpleasant symptoms may occur because it reduces the amount of carbon dioxide in the blood. This changes the balance of chemicals in the blood, causing tightening of the blood vessels and reduced blood supply, especially in the brain.

This reduced blood supply to the brain causes sensations such as light-headedness, dizziness, feeling faint, feeling unsteady, blurred vision, pins and needles, tingling, or numbness (sometimes one-sided) in the limbs or face, or clumsiness. Cramp-like muscle spasms may be experienced, particularly in the hands and feet. Increased sensitivity to light and noise may also occur, as well as abnormal sensations such as feelings of being detached from oneself. Feelings of unreality or being out of control may also occur.

Feelings of faintness are misleading, because blood pressure is usually high in times of anxiety and fainting occurs only when blood pressure is very low. However, anxiety may precede a faint when someone who has a blood and injury phobia has an injection or sees blood: in these situations, blood pressure drops, and fainting can occur.

The muscles of the chest wall can be overused during hyperventilation, which may lead to *chest pain* or *discomfort*. If these sensations are interpreted as signs of a serious problem, for example of heart trouble, that can lead to a further increase in anxiety and adrenaline production, leading to a further increase of unpleasant sensations.

Over-breathing also results in increased use of the muscles of the head, neck and shoulders, resulting in headaches and localised stiffness and pain.

Overuse of the neck muscles in hyperventilation can be accompanied by sensations of tightness or soreness in the throat.

Increased nerve activity and release of adrenaline may also cause excessive breathing through the mouth and reduced saliva production. These result in a dry mouth, swallowing difficulties and the feeling of a lump in the throat.

Altered blood flow

When we are anxious, blood is redirected to muscles to prepare for action. Reduced blood flow to the skin may cause *pallor, pain, coldness of hands and feet* and sometimes *numbness or tingling*.

Reduced blood flow to the bowel affects the passage of food and can result in *symptoms of irritable bowel*: for example, *constipation and/or diarrhoea and abdominal discomfort*.

Muscle tension

There is an increase in the tension of the muscles to prepare them for action.

This can cause aches, pains (particularly in the shoulders, neck, jaw and head) and fatigue. Muscular twitching or trembling may also occur.

Visual disturbance

Increased nerve activity affects the muscles of the iris (the coloured part of the eye), causing the pupils to dilate and so to let in more light. This may help to explain the sensitivity to bright light experienced by some people with CFS. The shape of the eye lens is altered to help improve side and distance vision. Together, the effects of these changes can be experienced as *blurring of vision.*

Sweating

Increased sweating occurs to allow for heat loss, causing *clammy hands and feet.*

Sleep disturbance

Adrenaline production increases at times of stress, so that sleep disturbance, for example *difficulty getting to sleep* or *frequent waking*, is very common; it may be accompanied by *nightmares* and *sweating*.

Mental functioning

Anxiety may affect mental functioning in a number of ways and contribute to the following:

- mood disturbance: for example, irritability, being easily upset;
- inability to concentrate, forgetfulness, indecisiveness;
- restlessness: for example, being fidgety or unable to sit still;
- a tendency to go over things again and again.

Everyone experiences physical symptoms of anxiety in an individual way, and few people have all of the symptoms listed above. However, when any of these symptoms are extreme, they can easily be misinterpreted as signs of a serious disease, and worry about this can trigger further unpleasant symptoms; this vicious circle can occasionally trigger a panic attack.

An increase in nerve activity and adrenaline production can precipitate feelings of weakness and exhaustion on top of the fatigue and muscle aches of chronic fatigue syndrome.

Management of chronic fatigue syndrome

Every person who has chronic fatigue syndrome has a different story to tell about what they have been advised to do by health professionals. This account will vary according to the beliefs or knowledge about CFS of the health-care professionals that you see; the availability of specialists in this area of medicine; and access to information about CFS: for example, through local support groups, the Internet, and so on.

You may feel that your illness has not been taken seriously. You may have been told that there is nothing wrong with you, that it is all in your mind, or that you should pull yourself together. On the other hand, you may have been told to rest until you feel better – or, conversely, to do as much as you can. You may have tried a number of remedies; or you may be reading this book without ever having talked to anyone about your chronic fatigue.

Even if a specific physical cause of your symptoms cannot be found, that does not mean there is nothing wrong with you. A combination of many factors may have precipitated and be maintaining your CFS. Every illness from the common cold to cancer can be affected by our lifestyle, attitudes, experiences and other things that happen around us. For example, you may have noticed that you are more likely to have a cold when you are particularly busy and under pressure.

In Part Two of this book we describe practical strategies to help you overcome your CFS. Some of the other treatments and remedies that are commonly used to help people with chronic fatigue syndrome are listed below.

Antidepressants

There is little evidence that antidepressants will reduce fatigue in people with chronic fatigue syndrome. However, they may be useful in treating any associated depression. Some antidepressants also contain properties that can alleviate muscle pain and insomnia.

Corticosteroids

There is not enough evidence of the effects of cortico-steroids in people with CFS to arrive at any conclusion about their usefulness. Any benefit from low doses has been short-lived, and higher doses have been linked with adverse effects such as adrenal suppression.

Immunotherapy

Again, there is a lack of substantial evidence to support the use of immunotherapy in people with CFS. Adverse effects, including headaches, fatigue and gastrointestinal disturbances, have been reported.

Dietary supplements

Little research has been carried out in this area. One study has shown benefits in some patients having magnesium injections. There have been mixed results from using evening primrose oil.

Diet

Various diets have been recommended in the treatment of chronic fatigue syndrome. If there is a proven allergy or intolerance, there may be benefits in excluding the aggra-vating food substance. Many people with CFS report being intolerant to alcohol and therefore exclude it from their diet. However, it is worth bearing in mind that avoiding any food for a while will result in a change in gastrointestinal functioning when reintroduced. Alterations in diet when travelling abroad, for example, may have similar effects.

Prolonged rest

Prolonged rest has not been shown to be helpful in the treatment of CFS. There is a lot of indirect evidence to suggest that prolonged rest may delay recovery because of the associated physical deconditioning.

Graded exercise

Graded exercise is designed to reverse the physical deconditioning (reduced fitness) and reduced muscle strength found in people who have chronic fatigue syndrome. It has been shown in several research trials to reduce fatigue and substantially improve physical functioning for people with CFS.

Pacing

Pacing is an energy-management strategy in which people with chronic fatigue syndrome are encouraged to achieve an appropriate balance between rest and activity. This usually involves living within the physical and mental limitations imposed by the illness and avoiding activities that exacerbate symptoms or interspersing activities with planned rests. The evidence for this is lacking, although pacing is helpful for those who tend to take on too much.

Complementary and alternative medicine

The terms 'complementary' and 'alternative' medicine refer to a wide range of approaches that aim to improve health and well-being. Although they are not generally considered to be part of mainstream medical care, they have been found helpful by people with a wide range of health problems and illnesses, including chronic fatigue syndrome. Although approaches including homoeopathy, osteopathy, acupuncture and herbal remedies have helped some people with CFS, there is no research evidence to support their use.

2

Understanding your own chronic fatigue problems

In order to understand your own fatigue problems better, it can be helpful to spend a bit of time thinking about when your own fatigue problems began and then to consider factors that may be contributing to keeping your fatigue going. Your own experience is unique and will include many factors we have described, as well as some that we haven't.

Understanding your own fatigue problems will help you to think about what might help you to get better.

Sarah's fatigue, for example, started when she was aged eighteen and studying for her A levels during the sixth form at school. She was feeling under pressure from the school and herself due to her own high standards. She was having difficulties with her boyfriend. Her situation made her feel a bit low and she also had a tendency to be anxious in social situations. During the next three years, her fatigue fluctuated and she particularly struggled when working part time and studying in her first year at university. In addition to fatigue, she had muscle pain in her arms and thighs and frequent headaches. She had difficulty in getting to sleep and felt unrefreshed in the morning. She had stopped going to the gym and doing yoga and was walking less. She was not attending all of her lectures and was behind on her reading. She was going out less with her friends and as a result of this was feeling increasingly anxious with people. She had moved home for her mum to look after her.

The fatigue experienced by Alison – a 43-year-old married woman with a ten-year-old son – began following a series of chest infections during a three-month period. She was working as a nursery nurse and didn't take time off as she did not want to let the children there down. She then developed flu during the Christmas holiday and rested a lot to help herself get better. When she tried to return to work in January, she felt exhausted and her limbs ached. Her memory and concentration were dramatically reduced, and she became distressed when she frequently forgot the names of children. After a couple of months, she gave up her job, feeling unable to cope. The next few years were very difficult for her. She spent a lot of time resting in the day but had difficulty sleeping at night. She tried to put on a brave face and be active when her son returned from school. She became less able to keep on top of the housework or cooking, and her husband became resentful, as he had to do these chores on return from a busy day at work. She began to feel demoralised, fearing that her once happy life was slipping away. Her circle of friends diminished, since she was less able to go out. Given that she was only able to walk short distances before feeling too weak to stand or walk, she reluctantly resorted to using a wheelchair away from home.

Ben's fatigue began after developing glandular fever during an extremely busy time in his life. He was twenty-three and had always been very fit and enjoyed running competitively. He would typically run up to sixty-five miles a week in ten or eleven sessions of varying distance and speed. He did well academically at school and obtained a 2:1 in a history degree before being employed on a graduation scheme. In February of the following year, he moved to a different work placement, which was stressful and where he worked long hours. He also moved house. He went on a skiing holiday in March and shared a room with someone who had glandular fever. He developed a sore throat and a cold. After a few days he felt a little better and ran a half-marathon, but felt unwell during it and had to walk the last few miles. The following week he had a vomiting bug and began to feel very fatigued. On return to work the following week, he felt exhausted and was unable to do anything in the evenings. He was signed off work for four consecutive months and on his return only managed four weeks before handing in his notice as he felt unable to continue. Once he stopped work, his fatigue improved a little, but he was unable to run for more than ten minutes at a time. He was prescribed three courses of antibiotics for his persistent sore throat; however, they did not improve his symptoms. He was seen by a physician in June, who diagnosed a likely Epstein-Barr virus (EBV), which is one of the most common human viruses.

The vicious cycle of fatigue

We often refer to factors that maintain fatigue as 'a vicious cycle', because one factor often leads to another that then reinforces the effect of the first, and so on. Figure 2.1 below demonstrates this. Although it is unlikely that it will completely fit your experience, you may be able to identify with some of it.

CONTRIBUTING FACTORS TO FATIGUE

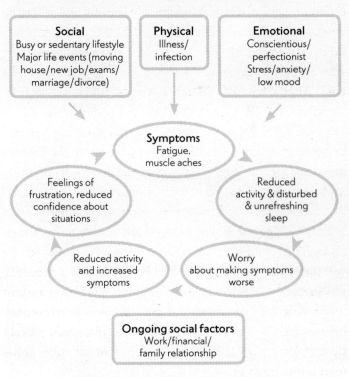

Figure 2.1 A vicious cycle of fatigue

SARAH'S EXAMPLE OF FACTORS CONTRIBUTING TO THE ONSET AND MAINTENANCE OF HER FATIGUE

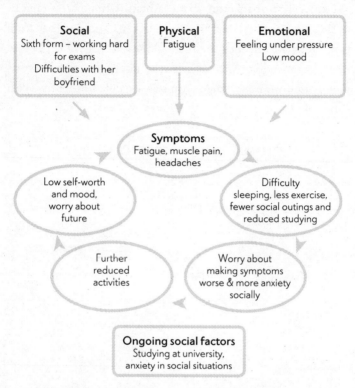

Figure 2.2 Sarah's vicious cycle of fatigue

There is space on page 35 for you to draw your own vicious cycle.

MY VICIOUS CYCLE OF FATIGUE

PART TWO

STEPS TO RECOVERY

Introduction

In this part of the book we aim to help you to tackle some of the things that may have been contributing to keeping your fatigue going. We hope that, as you try out the steps outlined here, your symptoms will become less intense or even go away; and that, if some of them do not, you will feel more confident to manage them, so that you will be able to do more of what you would like to do.

First, in Chapter 3, we talk about cognitive behavioural therapy (CBT) as a treatment for chronic fatigue syndrome. It is important that you know that the techniques included in this book have been used effectively to help people with CFS in research studies, by a variety of specially trained health professionals. We then outline what is involved in applying CBT techniques in a self-help programme designed to help overcome chronic fatigue.

3

Cognitive behavioural therapy for chronic fatigue

In this chapter, we briefly outline a few facts about cognitive behavioural therapy and how it has been used to help people. We then go through the steps that you will take on your journey. We would like you to pay particular attention to the short section on pages 49–53 titled 'A few words of warning!', as it will help you to clarify whether this is the right approach for you and whether you need to see your doctor before you make a start.

What is cognitive behavioural therapy?

Cognitive behavioural therapy is a 'talking' therapy that has been found to be valuable and effective in helping people with a variety of health problems that include chronic pain, irritable bowel syndrome and diabetes, as well as depression, eating disorders and anxiety. CBT is based on the principle that you can help manage your problems by changing the way you think (cognitive) and behave (behavioural).

Unfortunately, access to therapist-led CBT is not always available and, with this in mind, self-help programmes in the form of books, apps and web-based programmes have been developed. There is growing evidence that 'self-help' with minimal therapist contact can help people with a variety of problems. There is a list of recommended books published on the NHS website for people with a variety of problems, many of which are part of the Overcoming series. (Please see the front of this book for a list of problems tackled by the series.)

This book offers a 'self-help' programme that aims to help you to overcome your symptoms of chronic fatigue by following strategies that we have designed according to the principles of CBT and used in our professional therapy practice.

Although many people have been helped to overcome many different illnesses and disorders by using these self-help programmes, there are some people for whom they are not appropriate; so again, we urge you to read and consider the section 'A few words of warning!' before you embark on the work set out in the following chapters.

Has any research shown that CBT is helpful in CFS?

The effectiveness of CBT in treating CFS has been evaluated in many well-conducted research studies undertaken since the 1990s. Randomised controlled trials involve more than one treatment group. Participants are randomly assigned to a group and, after treatment, the groups are compared on a health outcome. In the case of CFS, the outcomes are usually measurements of fatigue and physical functioning. In previous studies CBT was found to produce better results than the other treatments with which they were compared. Graded exercise therapy is similarly effective. Although CBT may include some exercise, normal activity is usually the focus.

Steps to helping you get better

Chapters 4 to 14 will guide you through the steps you need to take to help you towards feeling better.

Please see the diagram on the next page, which illustrates the steps you will be taking on your journey towards reducing your fatigue and feeling better.

1. **Monitor your activity and sleep patterns**
   The first step involves you keeping activity diaries and sleep diaries for a few weeks. This information will help you to take a step back and see how your fatigue is affecting you day to day. It will also help you to create your first programme of planned activity and rest.

Activity diaries

We will ask you to keep an activity diary of what you are doing each day to help you to get an accurate picture of the

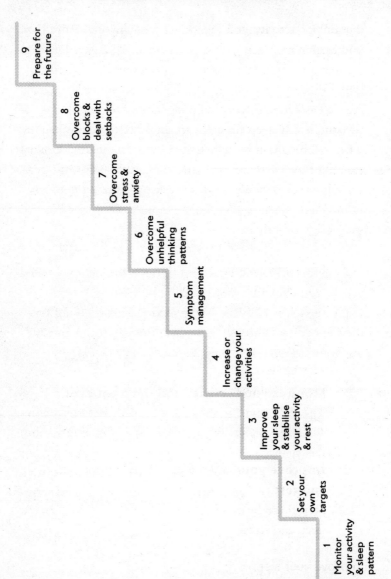

1 Monitor your activity & sleep pattern

2 Set your own targets

3 Improve your sleep & stabilise your activity & rest

4 Increase or change your activities

5 Symptom management

6 Overcome unhelpful thinking patterns

7 Overcome stress & anxiety

8 Overcome blocks & deal with setbacks

9 Prepare for the future

amount of activity you are doing and the amount of rest you are having.

Sleep diaries

As well as keeping an activity diary, we will be asking you to complete a sleep diary simultaneously for a few weeks. This will help you to get a general sense of your sleep pattern. You will also be able to see potential problem areas, such as taking a long time to go to sleep, waking frequently in the night, or sleeping for many hours on some nights and only a few on others, etc.

2. **Set your own targets**

   Step two involves you setting your own targets to help you to focus on what *you* would like to work towards during the next few months. It will give you the opportunity to think about targets that may help you to have a more enjoyable and better-balanced life. It is therefore a good idea to consider having targets across a range of areas of life – including social and leisure activities as well as work and home.

3. **Improve your sleep and stabilise your activity and rest**

   Step three helps you to learn ways to improve your sleep and stabilise your activities.

Improve your sleep

You will read about some practical things that you can do

to help improve the quality of your sleep. The strategies that you decide to use will depend on your specific sleep problem(s). For example, if you have no set times for going to bed or waking up, you may find it helpful to learn how to establish a routine. If you have problems falling asleep at night, you will learn ways to get to sleep more quickly: these may involve developing a routine before going to bed to increase your sleepiness, reducing sleep in the day and learning to cope with worries that may be keeping you awake.

Stabilise your activity and rests

If you have noticed from your diaries that you have a tendency towards an erratic pattern of activity and rest, then this section will be helpful. You will be asked to plan a programme of scheduled activity and rest, which you will review and change every week or so. The aim will be to try to carry out the same amount of activity and rest each day, in order to avoid 'bursts of activity' when feeling less fatigued or long periods of rest when more fatigued. Introducing short periods of relaxation will be important if you generally do too much.

4. Increase or change your activities

Once you have established more of a routine of activity and rest, you will be in a good position to work towards your targets. This may involve you gradually increasing some activities (e.g. walking, seeing friends or studying) and introducing new activities (e.g. doing a course, voluntary work or introducing a new form of exercise such as swimming). For some people, changing activity levels may mean reducing the time on certain activities e.g. shortening hours at work, particularly if working very long hours, or choosing to reduce time spent on chores.

5. Symptom management

In this step, we discuss a way to help you deal with unpleasant symptoms that you may be experiencing. Although doing things such as improving your sleep pattern and having a more consistent pattern of activity and rest may help to reduce some of your symptoms, the suggested strategy may provide you with further benefit.

6. Overcome unhelpful thinking patterns

The sixth step will help you to see how the way we think about things influences how we feel (emotionally and physically). How we think also affects how we behave or what we do. Initially you will be asked to identify thoughts that may be hampering your progress – e.g., 'I will feel exhausted if I go out for a walk' – or that make you feel frustrated, such as 'I'll never get better' or 'I used to be able to do so much more.' In time, you may find that you can be more objective about your thoughts i.e. see them as thoughts, not facts. You will learn how to challenge these thoughts by coming up with more helpful alternatives. If you find that you are having a number of thoughts around a similar theme, such as being self-critical, and that they are not going away when you try to challenge them, you will have the opportunity to deal with them by identifying and challenging deeper thoughts that we call 'core beliefs'.

7. Overcome stress and anxiety

Step six will hopefully have helped you to be able to challenge thoughts that make you feel anxious or stressed. This next step will help you to identify other ways to reduce or overcome stress or anxiety that you may be experiencing. It includes problem solving and learning to gradually face situations that you may not have faced for a while or that you want to face in order to achieve some of your targets.

8. Overcome blocks to recovery and deal with setbacks

Overcoming an illness is hardly ever straightforward. There may be times when you feel that you are doing everything you can to move forward, but you just don't seem to be making any progress. Chapter 11, on 'Overcoming blocks to recovery', outlines a number of 'blocks' that can make it more difficult for you to make progress and offers some suggestions on how you can overcome them. The next chapter then discusses how to manage setbacks; by this we mean when your symptoms suddenly increase for a few days or more and you find it harder to manage your activities. You will learn how to recognise triggers of setbacks and how to implement strategies to overcome these difficult times and move forward.

9. **Prepare for the future**
   Our final step is aimed at helping you to consolidate and reflect on all of your hard work, and then to plan how you are going to continue in order to maintain your progress and build on your gains.

A few words of warning!

Because we really want you to get as much out of this book as you can, we would like you to take a few minutes to consider the following points before you make a start on the steps outlined.

- **Make an appointment to see your doctor about your fatigue if you have not done so already.**
  We would expect that most people who read this book will already have seen their doctor to discuss their fatigue problem and, indeed, your doctor may have recommended that you might benefit from reading this book. If you have not, we strongly recommend that you do make an appointment before you start working through the self-help programme. Your doctor is likely to take a history of your symptoms and may suggest you have a few blood tests and possibly a urine test to rule out other diagnoses that may explain your symptoms.

49

- **Start working through the book when you can commit to it for some time.**

  We would recommend that you start working through this book when you feel able to commit to following its guidelines for a period of a few months. By doing this you are more likely to benefit. A lot of the strategies discussed in this book can take some time to master, and you may need to persevere with them for a while before feeling any better. If you have a lot of extra things going on in your life, such as being about to start exams, moving house, or looking after your children in the holidays, it may be best to wait for a calmer period of your life. It can be helpful to view this book as a course into which you have to invest time and effort to gain something from it.

- **Consider involving someone to offer you support.**

  Some people find it helpful to involve a partner, relative or close friend to help them work through this book. Having the support of a close person along the way can make a positive difference and may encourage you to keep going, particularly when things feel a little difficult. Chapter 15 on pages 303–311 provides some guidelines about how they may be able to help you.

- **Do not try other treatments while working through this book unless recommended by your doctor.**
  We would suggest that, unless recommended by your doctor, you do not try other new treatments to help your fatigue at the same time as working through this book. Starting more than one thing at a time can be confusing, as you may not know what specifically is helping you.

- **Be aware that your fatigue and other symptoms may temporarily increase.**
  Your fatigue and other symptoms may temporarily increase when you start your activity programme and/or when you introduce or increase activities; this is quite normal, and the symptoms should subside again after a short while.

- **When to see your doctor.**
  In the unlikely event that you experience a sudden or severe increase in your symptoms or begin to experience new symptoms that you have not noticed before, you should consult your doctor.

- **Persevere with your programme.**
  At times you may find the steps of the programme outlined in this book to be challenging. This is understandable, as you will have been doing things in your own way to manage your fatigue to the best

of your ability. As you will be aiming to do things at *regular* times, i.e. more consistently, there may be times when you feel frustrated that you cannot do what you *feel* like doing. For example, sometimes you may feel like resting for longer than your programme says, and at other times you may want to continue with a specific activity when the programme you have written says that you are meant to be resting. This is understandable! However, we would recommend that as far as possible you persevere with your programme. In time, you will appreciate the benefits of gradually changing the way you do things.

- **How to deal with a setback.**
  During the course of the programme, you may notice the odd minor setback, by which we mean an increase in your symptoms that lasts for a few days or so. This is very common, and we find that most people experience one or two setbacks during their course of CBT. Setbacks may come about for a variety of reasons, but are more likely when you have a viral infection or when there are additional stressful things going on in your life. The important thing is not to panic!

  Chapter 12 offers some guidelines on managing setbacks. Although these episodes may be worrying and frustrating, they can give you the opportunity to learn more about your own triggers to a setback, and help you to become an expert in managing difficult times.

Programme – Table of steps and actions

The programme outlined below is generally followed by people who attend CBT sessions with a therapist. However, it is possible to do this at home without a therapist. Unfortunately, it is not possible to give you firm guidelines on how long each step will take, as everyone is different! The important thing is that you work through at a pace that is comfortable to you. You may find that some parts are more relevant to you and you want to spend longer on them. There may be times when you are working through the book and feel unable to follow the guidelines for a while due to life events unexpectedly getting in the way. It is absolutely fine to put it aside for a short while and come back to it when you feel able to proceed again.

Programme – Table of steps and actions

STEP	ACTION	NOTES
Monitor your activity and sleep pattern	Read Chapter 4 Complete activity and sleep diaries	For 2–4 weeks
Set your targets	Read Chapter 5 Write targets to work towards	After completing diaries for a couple of weeks Set further targets once you have achieved the first ones or have come up with new ideas
Improve your sleep and stabilise your activity and rest	Read Chapter 6 and 7 Set your initial programme	When you have completed diaries for 2–4 weeks and are familiar with your sleep and activity patterns
Increase or change your activities	Read the relevant section in Chapter 7 Make changes to your initial programme	Once you have completed a more consistent pattern of activity and rest
Manage your symptoms	Read Chapter 8, pages 130–6	At a time of your choosing
Overcome unhelpful thinking patterns	Read Chapter 9 Identify and challenge unhelpful thinking patterns	If you are aware of troublesome thoughts and find that you are having difficulty making progress with your programme

Overcome stress and anxiety	Read Chapter 10	If life is stressful and hampering your progress
Overcome blocks and deal with setbacks	Read Chapter 11	If you feel stuck with your programme
	Read Chapter 12	If you notice that your symptoms are increasing for a few days or more
Prepare for the future	Read Chapter 13 and 14	A few months or so after starting your programme. When you have noticed some good improvement and achieved some of your targets

4

Monitoring activity, rest and sleep

This chapter describes how to monitor your waking and sleeping hours. We suggest keeping an activity diary in the daytime and a sleep diary for the night-time. For shift-workers, you can adapt the times in your diary to your 'waking' and 'sleeping' times. Keeping these records will help you to highlight specific patterns that may be contributing to keeping your fatigue going.

Monitoring your activity levels

To help you gain an accurate picture of how you spend each day, it is really important that you write down what you are doing in your activity diary.

We would recommend that you complete your activity diaries for at least two weeks. After a week or so, you may see a pattern emerging. For example, you may notice that you tend to be fairly active in the morning and rest all afternoon, or you may be busy during the week and do very little at the weekend. You may notice that you have short bursts of activity throughout the day, or you may not see any pattern at all.

After you are satisfied that the diaries you have completed are fairly typical of your routine, then it will be time for you to turn to Chapter 7 to plan your initial activity programme. For most people, this is after about two weeks. However, if you do not feel that the time over which you have been completing your diaries is typical, it may be wise to keep them going for another week or so. The reason for this is that the information from your activity diaries will help you to decide on how much rest and activity you should have each day.

What do I have to do?

- To help you understand what to write, please have a look at the three examples of completed activity diaries on pages 58–63.
- Photocopy the blank activity diary on pages 64–65, or if you would prefer to write your own timings down in the left-hand column, then use the one on the following pages 66–67.
- Write down every day (or during your waking hours) what you are doing at the times indicated in the left-hand column.
- Include what you were doing and for how long.
- Try to complete your diaries for every hour of the day, however trivial the activity may seem.
- Record your activities at regular intervals throughout the day.
- Turn to Chapter 7 when you feel ready to plan your first activity programme.

Activity diary, example 1: A person who rests for most of the time

Week beginning...................

DAY	MONDAY	TUESDAY	WEDNESDAY	THURSDAY	FRIDAY	SATURDAY	SUNDAY
Hours asleep last night	9 hours	10 hours	10½ hours	5 hours	9 hours	4¾ hours	7 hours
6–8 a.m.	Asleep	Asleep	Asleep	Asleep	Asleep	Woke at 6, dozed	Asleep
8–10 a.m.	Asleep	Woke at 9.30	Woke at 10	Woke at eight in pain	Woke at 9.30	Breakfast in bed	Woke at 8.15. Bath
10–11 a.m.	Took a bath and had breakfast	Breakfast in bed	Bath and dressed	Stayed in bed	Bath and dressed	Stayed in bed until lunch	Dressed and had breakfast
11 a.m.– 12 noon	Lay on the couch, resting	Washed face, brushed teeth	Doctor's appoint-ment	Slept	Rested on couch	Dozing	Went to friend's house
12 noon– 1 p.m.	Looked at paper	Lay on couch, read a letter	Home, exhausted	Mother brought up soup	Lunch	Dozing	Had lunch
1–2 p.m.	Lunch, made by Mum	Made toast and tea	To bed	Dozed	Shopping with Mum by car	Dressed, had lunch	Watched a video

Time							
2–3 p.m.	Went to bed and slept	Went to bed	Slept	Went downstairs	Watched television	Relations round	Went home (by car)
3–4 p.m.	Slept	Dozed on and off	Tea and toast in bed	Watched television	Tidied up (10 mins)		Lay on couch
4–5 p.m.	Went downstairs and watched TV	Friend came around	Went downstairs	Phoned a friend	Went to bed, feeling poorly		Dozed
5–6 p.m.			Lay on couch	Went back to bed	Slept	Felt exhausted; dozed on couch	Dozed
6–7 p.m.	Ate evening meal	Friend left, exhausted	Had evening meal	Evening meal in bed	Slept	Slept	Had a bath
7–8 p.m.	Television	Had evening meal	Television	Listened to radio	Evening meal downstairs	Evening meal	Evening meal in bed
8 p.m.–12 midnight	Bed at 10.15	Bed at 8.30	Bed at 9.15		Watched television	Friend phoned; television	Dozed on and off
Time I went to sleep	1 a.m.	11 p.m.	2 a.m.	12 midnight	2 a.m.	1.30 a.m.	

Activity diary, example 2: A person who manages some activity, but quite erratically

Week beginning.................

DAY	MONDAY	TUESDAY	WEDNESDAY	THURSDAY	FRIDAY	SATURDAY	SUNDAY
Hours asleep last night	7 hours	8 hours	8¼ hours	9 hours	6 hours	9½ hours	11 hours
6–8 a.m.	Woke at 8	Asleep	Asleep	Woke at 7, read in bed	Asleep	Asleep	Asleep
8–10 a.m.	Bath and dressed at 9	Up 8.45, bath and dressed	Dressed at 9.15, breakfast	Woke at 8, bath, dressed	Stayed in bed, felt rough	Got up at 10	Breakfast in bed
10–11 a.m.	Ate breakfast, washed up	Breakfast, tidied up	Walked to shops (15 mins)	Breakfast, cleared up	Slept	Bathed and dressed	Bath and dressed
11 a.m.–12 noon	Rested on couch	Bus to dentist	Unpacked shopping	Wrote a letter (½ hour)	Bath and dressed	Went to sister's house by train (1¾ hrs door to door)	Played with children
12 noon–1 p.m.	Lunch	Walked home (20 mins)	Lunch	Walked to post letter (10 mins)	Ate a sandwich		Went for a bar lunch
1–2 p.m.	Watched TV	Lunch	Rested on bed (dozing)	Lunch	Walked to shops (15 mins)	Played with sister's children	

2–3 p.m.	Walked to shops (15 mins)	Slept on couch		Friend visited; chatted	Met friend, went to her house	Walk in the park (25 mins)	Walked in park (½ hr)
3–4 p.m.	Rested		Tidied my room		Listened to music	Fell asleep on couch	Train home
4–5 p.m.	Rested	Read for fifteen mins	Read downstairs	Dozed on couch	Fell asleep	Helped to feed children	
5–6 p.m.	Cooked and ate evening meal	Watched TV	Visited friends	Watched TV	Walked home (15 mins)	Read children a story	Fell asleep on couch
6–7 p.m.	Washed up, read (5 mins)	Prepared and ate evening meal		Cooked and ate evening meal	Heated a pre-packed meal	Had a take-out	Made a sandwich
7–8 p.m.	Listened to the radio	Washed up		Washed up	Ate evening meal and washed up	Chatted to sister	Went to bed and read
8 p.m.–12 midnight	Friend visited	Phoned friend. Bed at 9.15	Home, bed immediately	Bad headache, bed at 8.30	Watched TV	Went to bed at 11	
Time I went to sleep	12.30 a.m.	1.30 a.m.	10 p.m.	11 p.m.	11.30 p.m.	11.05 p.m.	9.30 p.m.

61

Activity diary, example 3: A person who is working, but is managing to do little at weekends or in the evenings

Week beginning.............

DAY	MONDAY	TUESDAY	WEDNESDAY	THURSDAY	FRIDAY	SATURDAY	SUNDAY
Hours asleep last night	8 hours	7 hours	9 hours	6 hours	7 hours	11 hours	11 hours
6–8 a.m.	Woke at 8	Up 6.30. 2-hour drive to London	Asleep	Woke at 7, had shower	Up at 6.30	Asleep	Asleep
8–10 a.m.	Train to work	Breakfast, met clients	Woke at 8.30, had long bath	Train to work; paperwork	Train to work, then meetings	Asleep	Up at 9.45
10–11 a.m.	Meetings all morning	Met clients	Worked at home	Interviews all morning	Meetings	Asleep	Played with children
11 a.m.– 12 noon		Meetings for most of the day				Got up at 11.30	Did some gardening
12 noon– 1 p.m.						Lunch	Went to lunch with friends

62

MONITORING ACTIVITY, REST AND SLEEP

	1–2 p.m.	2–3 p.m.	3–4 p.m.	4–5 p.m.	5–6 p.m.	6–7 p.m.	7–8 p.m.	8 p.m.–12 midnight	Time I went to sleep
	Lunch at desk (10 mins)	Paperwork and phone calls				Train home; phone calls	Evening meal	Watched TV. Bed at 10	10.30 p.m.
	Lunch at restaurant				Drove home, took 3 hours		Evening meal	Fell asleep at about 8.30	8.30 p.m.
		Train to work	Paperwork	Phone calls	Meeting		Took clients out for a meal	Home at 11.30	1 a.m.
	Lunch at desk	Paperwork and phone calls			Home, read to children	Long relaxing bath	Evening meal	Work for tomorrow	1 a.m.
	Lunch out with colleagues		Paperwork	Phone calls	Train home	Friends round for evening meal		Bed at midnight	12.30 p.m.
	Watched sport on TV			Helped feed children	Read children a story	Fell asleep	Evening meal	Watched a video	11 p.m.
			Home, fell asleep		Prepared for meeting Monday	Long relaxing bath	Evening meal	More work. Bed at 11	12 midnight

Activity diary

Week beginning..................................

DAY	MONDAY	TUESDAY	WEDNESDAY	THURSDAY	FRIDAY	SATURDAY	SUNDAY
Hours asleep last night							
6–8 a.m.							
8–10 a.m.							
10–11 a.m.							
11 a.m.–12 noon							
12 noon–1 p.m.							
1–2 p.m.							

MONITORING ACTIVITY, REST AND SLEEP

2–3 p.m.	3–4 p.m.	4–5 p.m.	5–6 p.m.	6–7 p.m.	7–8 p.m.	8 p.m.–12 midnight	Time I went to sleep

Activity diary

Week beginning............

DAY	MONDAY	TUESDAY	WEDNESDAY	THURSDAY	FRIDAY	SATURDAY	SUNDAY
Hours asleep							

							Time I went to sleep

Monitoring your sleep pattern

To help you to build up an accurate picture of how you sleep, complete a sleep diary for two weeks. This will help you to see at a glance what your sleep pattern is like and any areas of difficulty that you are having. For example, you may notice that on some nights it takes you a while to get to sleep, that you get up at very different times each day or that you wake frequently in the night.

What do I have to do?

- Look at the example of a completed sleep diary on page 69.
- Photocopy the blank sleep diary on page 70 for your own use.
- Complete your sleep diary when you wake up in the morning for at least two weeks.
- After completing your sleep diary for two weeks, read Chapter 6, which outlines a number of strategies to help you to improve your sleep.
- Decide what you would like to change about your sleep pattern and, when you come to construct your first activity programme (Chapter 7), write down the strategies that will help you to achieve your aims.
- You may find it helpful to continue to keep a sleep diary for a few more weeks to see if your sleep improves as you implement some of the strategies.

Example of a completed sleep diary

Week beginning...........

	MON.	TUES.	WED.	THURS.	FRI.	SAT.	SUN.
Last night I went to bed at . . . and turned the lights out at . . .	9.15 p.m. 10 p.m.	9.30 p.m. 9.45 p.m.	10 p.m. 10.30 p.m.	9.45 p.m. 10.15 p.m.	11 p.m. 11 p.m.	12.30 a.m. 12.30 a.m.	9.30 p.m. 9.45 p.m.
After turning out the lights, I fell asleep in . . . (estimate)	30 mins	Straight away	Straight away	1 hour	5–10 mins	Straight away	About 2 hours
I woke up . . . times in the night	1	0	0	2	0	1	2
On each waking during the night, I was awake for . . . (estimate)	2 mins	–	–	5 mins 30 mins	–	5 mins	15 mins 30 mins
I woke up at . . . (time of last waking)	8 a.m. with alarm	7.30 a.m.	8 a.m. with alarm	9.30 a.m.	8 a.m. with alarm	10 a.m.	8.30 a.m.
I got out of bed for the day at . . .	8.30 a.m.	8 a.m.	8.15 a.m.	10 a.m.	8.15 a.m.	10.30 a.m.	9 a.m.
Overall, my sleep last night was . . . (0=very sound, 8=very restless)	2	0	0	5	0	2	2
When I got up this morning I felt . . . (0=refreshed, 8=exhausted)	5	4	4	6	3	5	6
Comments/reasons for a good or a particularly bad night				Felt hot and achy	Better night: bath before bed relaxed me		Worrying about interview tomorrow

69

Sleep diary

Week beginning................

	MON.	TUES.	WED.	THURS.	FRIDAY	SAT.	SUN.
Last night I went to bed at . . . and turned the lights out at . . .							
After turning out the lights, I fell asleep in . . . (estimate)							
I woke up . . . times in the night							
On each waking during the night, I was awake for . . . (estimate)							
I woke up at . . . (time of last waking)							
I got out of bed for the day at . . .							
Overall, my sleep last night was . . . (0=very sound, 8=very restless)							
When I got up this morning I felt . . . (0=refreshed, 8=exhausted)							
Comments/reasons for a good or a particularly bad night							

5

Setting targets

Setting targets is an important step in helping you to over-come your chronic fatigue problems and an opportunity to identify things that you would like to do that would give your life more meaning or value. In the past, you may have prioritised just a few activities such as work and looking after the family, and may have neglected time for yourself – your hobbies or interests, time to see your friends, and so on. Setting targets will therefore give you the opportunity to develop a more 'balanced' lifestyle that includes more of the things that you *want* to do rather than just the things that you feel that you *should* do. This in turn can contribute to reducing your fatigue and helping you to feel generally happier and more fulfilled.

Pie charts

In order to work out how 'balanced' your life feels, it can be helpful to think about what your life looks like in terms of a pie chart. By this we mean examine all aspects of your life such as sleep, work, study, exercise, interests/hobbies, relaxation, relationship, childcare, social, etc. and allocate a proportion of time to each.

You could look at what your life looks like now in 'Pie chart A' and then think about how you would like things to be in 'Pie chart B'. It may help you to come up with some targets that you would like to work towards.

When you compare pie chart A and B below, you can see that this person decided to slightly reduce their work/study time, do less chores and slightly increase 'time for me' and sleep.

Pie Chart (A)

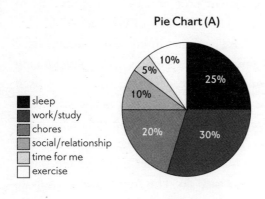

Pie Chart (B)

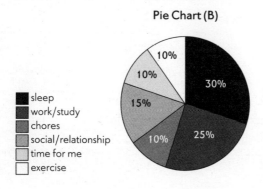

We have left two blank pie charts for you to complete on the next two pages.

Pie Chart (A)

- Use the lines below to write out what your life *currently* looks like.
- Use the pie chart to divide your activities into segments.

_____

_____

_____

_____

_____

_____

_____

_____

Pie Chart (B)

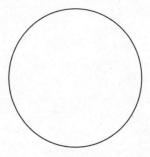

Use the space below to write out how you would like your life to look. For example, if you have noticed in your first pie chart that there are areas missing or too much or too little time spent on certain activities, then think about changes you would like to make.

Using this information, write down changes on your pie chart that you want to make and apportion a percentage to it.

_____

_____

_____

_____

_____

_____

_____

_____

When would be a good time to plan my targets?

We suggest that you set a few targets at the same time that you plan your first activity programme. This could be after completing your activity and sleep diaries for two to four weeks. In addition to completing your pie charts, keeping activity and sleep diaries can help you to identify areas of your life that you would like to change. As you proceed through the chapters of this book, you may identify other targets that you would like to work towards; you can add new ones at any time.

Important facts about targets

- Targets are things that you would like to be doing in the longer term, rather than things you want to achieve immediately.
- Set yourself a range of *different* types of targets to work towards, taking into consideration responsibilities as well as things that would make your life more enjoyable, enriching and balanced. So, rather than addressing one specific area of your life, e.g. work or studying, try to ensure that your targets contain a *mixture* of activities.
- Remember that pleasurable activities and time for you are as important as income-earning work, household chores, etc.
- Set yourself *realistic* and *achievable* targets. Be wary

of being too 'driven' or 'ambition-orientated' when setting your targets. For example, if you have not worked for several years, it would be better to set yourself a target of taking up voluntary or part-time work, rather than a full-time job. Or, if you have not walked much for a long time, it is important to set moderate targets such as walking for fifteen minutes a day. Remember that you will be able to add new targets once your initial ones have been achieved; you shouldn't bite off more than you can chew at the first attempt.

- Make your targets *specific*, in terms of:
  1. *what it is* you want to do (activity);
  2. *how often* you would like to carry out the activity (frequency);
  3. the *length of time* to be spent on the activity (duration).

- Although you may feel that your choice of targets is restricted because of your symptoms, setting targets, however modest, will provide you with a clear direction and focus.

- You may need to enlist the help of a partner, other family member or friend to be able to achieve some of your targets. For example, if you decide that you are doing the majority of chores at home and want to work towards more social activities or relaxation time for yourself, you could discuss with family members the idea of delegating some of the chores to them.

Please see below the targets that Alison planned to work towards in the longer term:

- To walk twice daily for twenty minutes.
- To cook a meal every night.
- To attend an evening/day class once a week.
- To go out with friends once a week for up to two hours.

How to set targets

- Look at the examples of target areas on the next two pages.
- Write a list of things that you would like to work towards over the coming months.
- Divide your list into target areas (e.g. work, social, exercise, leisure).
- Look at the examples of targets on pages 80–2, to ensure that your targets are clearly defined and specific.
- Choose at least four targets. You may find it helpful to break each target into manageable steps using a target breakdown sheet, as described on pages 82–5. Blank sheets are provided on pages 86–8.

Examples of target areas

Leisure time

- You may find that your time at home is taken up with chores. Think about planning regular time for pleasurable activities; for example, reading, playing a musical instrument, doing puzzles, reading your favourite book or paper. Write a poem, story or song, write each day in a diary, draw or paint a picture, knit, sew or crochet. Do a puzzle with a lot of pieces or a Sudoku or crossword. Change your hair colour or have a hair-cut. Have a massage. Have 'quality time' with children or partner. Plan a half or full day to go somewhere new. Cook your favourite dish or meal or try a new recipe. Enrol in a short course of something that you would find interesting or fun (pottery, art, music, language, etc.).

Exercise

In the past, you may have exercised regularly or played a sport. On the other hand, you may never have been particularly fit and have had exercise on a 'to-do' list for many years. You may like to consider setting aside time for regular exercise; it doesn't have to be anything strenuous: walking has many benefits! Not only is regular exercise known to be good for physical and mental health and good sleep quality, but results from a recent study indicated that carrying out a small amount of walking a day, and building up gradually, improved fatigue and physical functioning.

Work/education

If you are *not* working, you may consider going back to your old job (if applicable), doing part-time work, or doing some voluntary work. If you *are* working, you may feel that you are working excessively, and would benefit from changing your job or reducing your hours.

You may consider some type of educational course to enable you to find work or change direction in your career. Alternatively, you may simply want to develop a new interest. The material in Chapter 14 on work, courses and resources (see pages 288–98) may provide you with some useful leads.

Social activities

There may be friends and family with whom you have lost touch, or who you see only rarely. You may like to consider making a regular time for talking to, emailing or meeting up with those people. Alternatively, you may like to explore options for meeting new people such as joining a club.

DIY/gardening/chores

DIY/gardening

You may have been unable to do much in your home or garden for some time because of your fatigue and may feel that you would like to work towards building in time for specific DIY or gardening projects. For example, buy plants for your garden and plant them, work on your bike or car, paint a room, build a rockery, etc.

Chores

You may feel that you are endlessly doing chores to try to maintain the 'high' standards you set yourself before becoming fatigued. If this is the case, you may choose to cut the time that you spend on the activity or delegate chores to other family members (if applicable). On the other hand, if, because of your fatigue, you have reduced or stopped an activity such as cooking, taking children to school, etc., you may choose to reintroduce this as a target.

Sleep

If sleep is a big problem, you may choose to focus on a specific target in relation to this; for example, a regular getting-up time, or not sleeping in the day.

Examples of clearly defined targets

- To go shopping twice a week for half an hour.
- To have a friend for coffee once a week for half an hour.
- To walk for fifteen minutes daily.
- To do voluntary work three times a week for at least two hours on each occasion.
- To go out with friends once a week for up to three hours.
- To swim twice weekly for half an hour on each occasion.

- To do a course at college for three hours weekly.
- To have a relaxing bath for half an hour three times weekly.
- To spend one hour daily on my hobby (specify the hobby).
- To do one hour of chores five times weekly: e.g. ironing, washing, cleaning.
- To work part time for at least two days per week.
- To cook a meal using fresh ingredients three times weekly.
- To go on five-kilometre park runs every Saturday.
- To help my children with their homework and/or play with them for half an hour daily.
- To have two breaks at work of at least fifteen minute each, daily.
- To sit and read the paper/a magazine for half an hour daily.
- To get up by 8:00 a.m. each day.
- To stay out of bed until 10 p.m. each night.

These are all measurable targets, so you will know when you have achieved them.

Examples of not clearly defined targets

- To go back to work. (No frequency or duration specified.)
- To go out socially more often. (No frequency or duration specified.)

- To be more active. (No activity, frequency or duration specified.)
- To get up earlier. (No activity, frequency or duration specified.)

These are just vague ideas and not measurable; you would therefore not know when you had met them, and would risk feeling uncertain, frustrated and discouraged about your progress.

How to break down your targets into manageable steps

As we have already mentioned, targets are things that you want to achieve in the longer term. Therefore, in order to work towards them in such a way that you can monitor your progress, you may find it helpful to break down each one into manageable steps. You can then gradually introduce the consecutive steps into your activity programme.

- Look at the examples below that have been broken down into manageable steps.
- Think of ways to break down each of your own targets into manageable chunks.
- Make each step small, and grade it from easy to difficult.
- Write down your steps to achieving your targets on your target breakdown sheets (see pages 86–8 for some blank sheets).

Examples of breaking down targets into manageable steps

Target: To go for two ten-minute walks every day.

STEPS TO ACHIEVING TARGET:

- To get out of bed/up from my chair each hour and walk round the room.
- To walk round my house for one minute every hour.
- To walk round the garden/house for two minutes each hour.
- To go for three three-minute walks every day.
- To go for three five-minute walks every day.
- To go for two seven-minute walks every day.
- To go for two ten-minute walks every day.

Target: To go out with friends once a week for up to three hours.

STEPS TO ACHIEVING TARGET:

- To talk to a friend on the phone for fifteen minutes three times a week.
- To go to a friend who lives close by for half an hour once a week.
- To go to a friend who lives close by for an hour once a week.
- To go out with a friend to a local venue for an hour once a week.
- To go out with friend(s) for one and a half hours a week.

- To go out with friend(s) for two hours a week.
- To go out with friend(s) for two and a half hours a week.
- To go out with friend(s) for three hours a week.

Target: To read for half an hour, twice a day.

STEPS TO ACHIEVING TARGET:

- To read for fifteen minutes, twice a day.
- To read for twenty minutes, twice a day.
- To read for thirty minutes, twice a day.

Target: To do voluntary work three times a week for at least two hours on each occasion.

STEPS TO ACHIEVING TARGET:

- To write a list of kinds of voluntary work in which I am interested.
- To contact the appropriate association(s) for information.
- To plan steps that will help me *sustain* the activity in which I want to be involved: e.g. standing for longer periods (if working in a charity shop), reading/computer work (if doing administrative work), etc.
- Arrange informal visit(s) to the workplace.
- Arrange a graded work schedule if possible: e.g. one hour twice weekly for a couple of weeks; then one hour three times a week; then two hours three times a week.

Target: To do something relaxing for myself for one hour every day.

STEPS TO ACHIEVING TARGET:

- To leave work on time each day.
- To ask other family members to help with the chores.
- To make a list of non-urgent tasks that can be put off to another day.
- To plan a list of pleasurable things that I would like to do each day.
- To choose one of these each day and spend an hour on it.

You may only need two or three steps to achieve a target, or you may need a lot more. We have included space on each target breakdown sheet for two targets, with eight steps to each. Use extra paper if there is not enough space on the sheets for all the steps you want to include.

TARGET BREAKDOWN SHEET

TARGET	STEPS TO ACHIEVING TARGET
_____	1 _____
_____	2 _____
_____	3 _____
_____	4 _____
_____	5 _____
_____	6 _____
_____	7 _____
_____	8 _____
TARGET	STEPS TO ACHIEVING TARGET
_____	1 _____
_____	2 _____
_____	3 _____
_____	4 _____
_____	5 _____
_____	6 _____
_____	7 _____
_____	8 _____

TARGET BREAKDOWN SHEET

TARGET	STEPS TO ACHIEVING TARGET
_____	1 _____
_____	2 _____
_____	3 _____
_____	4 _____
_____	5 _____
_____	6 _____
_____	7 _____
_____	8 _____

TARGET	STEPS TO ACHIEVING TARGET
_____	1 _____
_____	2 _____
_____	3 _____
_____	4 _____
_____	5 _____
_____	6 _____
_____	7 _____
_____	8 _____

TARGET BREAKDOWN SHEET

TARGET	STEPS TO ACHIEVING TARGET
_____	1 _____
_____	2 _____
_____	3 _____
_____	4 _____
_____	5 _____
_____	6 _____
_____	7 _____
_____	8 _____
TARGET	STEPS TO ACHIEVING TARGET
_____	1 _____
_____	2 _____
_____	3 _____
_____	4 _____
_____	5 _____
_____	6 _____
_____	7 _____
_____	8 _____

6

Improving your sleep

Sleep problems in people with chronic fatigue are very common. Difficulties include:

- taking a long time to go to sleep at night;
- waking frequently and/or staying awake during the night;
- waking early;
- sleeping too much.

The quality of sleep is often poor and often results in waking up unrefreshed or feeling exhausted.

This chapter aims to help you to identify some of the things that may be contributing to your sleep problems (if applicable) and offers strategies to overcome each one.

When would be a good time to implement the suggested strategies?

You can begin to implement the suggested strategies after you have been keeping your sleep diary for a couple of weeks. By this time, you will have had a chance to identify patterns and what you want to change. You may introduce some changes to your sleep routine at the same time as you construct your first activity programme.

We have included a variety of strategies to try, depending on your own problems and targets in relation to sleep. Please do not feel that you need to implement them all at once, as you may feel overwhelmed by trying to change too many things too quickly. So, for example, if you stay in bed until lunchtime every day, and have a nap in the afternoon, and go to bed in the early evening, you may find it easier to start by gradually getting up earlier and cutting out or reducing the nap, while leaving your bedtime the same. You can decide what works best for you in terms of *how* you work on each sleep-related target. So, for example, if you are currently getting up at around 12 noon and have set a longer-term target to get up by 8:00 a.m. you may prefer to aim to get up earlier by an amount of time that feels sustainable to you, such as half an hour to an hour. Some people do opt for a radical change to try to achieve their target more quickly; however, this can substantially increase fatigue for a while!

- Write down the strategies that you intend to use to work towards your sleep-related targets on your activity programme. A blank one for you to photocopy can be found on page 126.

Lifestyle and environmental factors that contribute to poor sleep

- *An irregular sleep pattern* can disrupt the body clock

and lead to the loss of certain cues, such as feeling tired in the evening and alert in the morning. For more information about this, please refer to Chapter 1, pages 17–20.

- *Daytime inactivity* can increase your feeling of fatigue and desire for sleep in the day.
- *Sleeping in the day* for more than a few minutes is likely to make it harder for you to fall asleep at night.
- *Alcohol and other substances*, such as caffeine-containing drinks (coffee, tea, cola), cigarettes and certain medications can make it difficult to go to sleep and/or wake you up in the night.
- *An uncomfortable sleeping environment*, such as being too hot or cold, a restless partner, excessive noise, or an uncomfortable mattress, may keep you awake at night.
- Activities in your bed or bedroom such as *studying, eating, using your phone or computer* may make it more difficult for you to fall asleep, as you may associate your bed or bedroom with daytime activity and have difficulty in 'switching off'.
- *Long periods of wakefulness* in bed may also lead you to associate your room or bed with being awake, therefore making it more difficult for you to go to sleep.
- *An overly active mind or worries at bedtime* can lead to tension, restlessness and an inability to relax, again making it more difficult to fall asleep.
- *Sleeping too much* can make you feel like you've got a hangover or are jet-lagged! This is because when you

sleep too much, you are throwing off your 'biological clock' that controls your circadian rhythms, which in turn can induce a sense of fatigue.

Strategies to improve your sleep

We have included a variety of strategies to help you with your own individual sleep problem. You may find that some work better than others for you. It may take a few weeks or so for you to notice much change in your sleep, but do persevere, as improving your sleep is likely to improve your feelings of fatigue.

Establish a routine of getting up at the same time each day

The aim of establishing a routine of getting up at a regular time is to help your body clock to get used to certain things happening at set times. This will help to regulate your body (circadian) rhythms. You will begin to 'feel' things, such as sleepiness at certain times each day and a regular sleep–wake cycle will be established. We do not recommend that you start out by going to bed at the same time every evening, as you may not feel sleepy. However, you may eventually find that when you start getting up at the same time each day you get sleepy at a particular time in the evening, and therefore naturally start going to bed at a similar time.

The guidelines below will help you to establish a routine. If your sleep pattern is very erratic, you may find it difficult to put them into practice all at once, and if this is the case, introduce them gradually

In order to establish a routine:

- *Try to get up at the same time each day*, even if you have not had much sleep the previous night. It may be helpful to set your alarm clock. If you tend to sleep through alarms, get a louder one. If you wake up and hit the snooze button and fall back to sleep, then try moving the alarm to the other side of the room so that you have to get out of bed. Some people find asking someone to wake them or phone them at their planned getting-up time helpful.
- *Try not to nap in the day* for longer than fifteen to twenty minutes, even if you feel very tired, as this is likely to disrupt your sleep at night. If this is too difficult, then gradually reduce the duration of your nap(s).
- *Try not to go to bed too early*, even if you feel very tired, or to make up for lost sleep. You may find it helpful to set a time before which you will **not** go to bed.

Associate your bed and bedroom with sleep rather than being awake

If you have slept badly over a long period of time or spent a lot of time in bed during the day, you may find that when you get into bed at night, you feel wide awake or restless, and cannot fall asleep easily. Subconsciously, you may therefore associate your bed/bedroom with being awake rather than being asleep and this in itself may make it harder to fall asleep.

The following guidelines aim to help you to associate your bed and bedroom with sleep rather than wakefulness.

- Avoid using your bedroom during the day if at all possible. If, however, you live in a one-room apartment, or one room in a house or student accommodation, try to have a separate work area in your room, so that you just use your bed for sleep.

- Your bed should be for sleep and (if applicable) sex only. So, try not to read, study, eat, watch television, use your computer or phone, or sort out the day's problems in bed, as these are waking activities. If this is not practical, e.g., if you do not have something else comfy to sit on in your room, then try to change the bed when you are not sleeping by putting a cover and possibly cushions on it. You can then use your bed in the day, but sit on it rather than getting in it. When you are ready for sleep, you can take off the cushions and pull down the cover. This action will help you to associate your bed with sleep rather than waking activities.

- Go to bed when you are sleepy, rather than at a time you think you should go. For example, if you think that you should go to bed at about 11.00 p.m., but do not feel sleepy, wait until you feel sleepy, as this is likely to speed up the process of falling asleep.

- Do not be tempted to go to bed very early (e.g. before 9:30 p.m.), even if you feel very sleepy, as you may wake up in the middle of the night or very early in the morning and have difficulty falling asleep again.

- Turn the light off straight away when you get into bed.

- If you are not asleep within about twenty minutes, go to another room and sit and relax or read until you feel sleepy again. It may be helpful to have the room pre-prepared, for example, with a book or magazine, music and a warm cover; this will help you to relax more quickly and will also increase the likelihood that you will get out of bed if unable to sleep. If you do not have another room to go to, then try to sit in a chair or on a bean bag, relaxing as described above until you feel sleepy.

- Repeat the previous step as often as is required, and also if you wake up for periods of more than about twenty minutes in the night.

Try to follow this programme as strictly as you can, as it can really help you to fall asleep and stay asleep. You may need to persevere with these steps for a while until you notice an improvement. If you have a partner, you may like to discuss with them ways that they can help you to keep to these guidelines. This may involve some compromises for both of you; for example, neither of you watching television in bed, or both aiming to go to bed at a similar time.

Establish an optimal sleep pattern

An optimal sleep pattern is one in which you fall asleep within a short time of going to bed, have good-quality sleep and wake seldom and only briefly, if at all, during the night.

Your sleep pattern is *optimal* when it is both *efficient* and *regular*. When you are asleep for the greater proportion of the time you spend in bed, the more *efficient* your sleep is. The more closely one night's time in bed and time asleep resemble other nights', the more *regular* your sleep is. To establish your optimal sleep pattern, you will reduce the amount of time you are in bed in order to increase the amount of time you are asleep. This can be done in conjunction with the guidelines in the above two sections, or separately.

If you sleep too much, reduce your sleep at night

As we have already mentioned, sleeping for longer than you need can result in feeling exhausted in the morning. So, if you are sleeping for an hour or more longer than you used to before having CFS, you may feel better if you reduce the amount of time you sleep at night.

- Cut down your sleep time gradually, either by going to bed half an hour later or by getting up half an hour earlier.
- Be consistent in either getting up earlier or going to bed later.

- Try not to compensate by getting up later or going to bed earlier, even if you feel more tired.
- Review your sleep diary weekly and continue to reduce your sleep time until you have reached your pre-CFS amount of sleep or feel more 'refreshed' on waking.

You may feel more tired at first after reducing your sleep at night, but in the long run you can expect the quality of your sleep to improve as the quantity of your sleep decreases.

Improve your sleep hygiene

'Sleep hygiene' refers to lifestyle and environmental factors that may be beneficial or detrimental to sleep.

The following guidelines may help to promote an improved sleep pattern.

- *Exercise:* There is evidence that exercise in the late afternoon can deepen your sleep at night. However, avoid strenuous exercise within three hours of bedtime, as this may wake you up.
- *Exposure to natural daylight:* Try to go outside during daylight because exposure to sunlight during the day and having darkness at night can help to maintain a healthy sleep–wake cycle.
- *Diet:* A light snack before bedtime may be sleep-inducing, but a heavy or rich meal too close to bedtime may interfere with your sleep.

- *Fluid intake* should be limited within an hour or two of going to bed to reduce the need to visit the bathroom.

- *Caffeine* stimulates the central nervous system; it is associated with delaying sleep onset and can cause wakefulness. Substances containing caffeine – e.g. coffee, tea, chocolate and cola – should be avoided for four to six hours before bedtime and during the night if you wake up. Coffee generally contains about twice as much caffeine as other caffeinated drinks.

- *Nicotine* also stimulates the central nervous system, and although many people say that cigarettes help them to relax, the overall effect is one of stimulation rather than relaxation. Smoking cigarettes should therefore be avoided near bedtime and if you wake in the night.

- *Alcohol* depresses the central nervous system. Although it may help you to drop off to sleep, after a few hours it acts as a stimulant, increasing the number of awakenings and generally decreasing the quality of sleep at night. It is unusual for people with CFS to drink much alcohol, as they often report increased sensitivity to it, but, if you do, it is best avoided three hours before bedtime and try to stick to only one or two drinks. A milky drink before bed can help you to feel sleepy and will not cause you to wake in the night.

- *Environment:* Your bed, mattress and pillow(s) should be comfortable. Keep light and noise to a minimum during your sleep period. Don't keep your bedroom too hot – it should be around 18° C. Use window blinds if necessary, earplugs if you live in a particularly noisy place and are unable to get used to it, and a fan or heater to control temperature.

Preparing for sleep

Establishing a set routine will help you to prepare both mentally and physically for going to sleep.

- Try to wind down in the hour or so before you go to bed.
- Include relaxing activities such as watching television, having a warm bath, listening to music in your 'winding-down' schedule.
- Avoid stimulating activities that will keep you alert: e.g. work, studying, using your computer or phone, or making difficult decisions. Some people also find watching television to be stimulating.
- Develop a regular order of doing things e.g. locking up the house, turning out the lights, brushing your teeth. This will act as a signal to your body that it is preparing for sleep and may increase feelings of sleepiness.

Problem-solving strategy for reducing worries at night

Lying in bed at night worrying about problems can make us all feel tense and make it harder to fall asleep. It can really help if you address worries during the day to allow your mind to relax and 'switch off' in bed. The strategy described below may help you to get to sleep more quickly.

- Set aside fifteen to twenty minutes in the early evening.
- Use this time to write down problems or loose ends that you have not had time to deal with during the day. (Please see example on the next page.)
- Write down one or two possible steps to resolve the problem(s).
- Allocate time to put your plans into action, e.g., the following day, as knowing when you are going to address the problems may also help to put your mind at rest.
- Also consider other, longer-term problems that may intrude on your sleep e.g. emotional, financial or any other worries.
- For each of these, write down the first or next positive step of action to take, and when you will take it.
- If you feel that there is nothing in particular that is worrying you or likely to keep you awake, then use the time to do something relaxing for you!
- Once you are in bed, if you cannot go to sleep or wake up worrying about a problem, remind yourself that you have the matter in hand and that worrying about it now will not help.
- If new worries occur to you at night, write them down on a notepad or a piece of paper, and 'deal'

with them the next day, in the ways described above.

- You may also find it helpful to refer to Chapter 10 on 'Overcoming worry, stress and anxiety related to your chronic fatigue', and Chapter 9 on 'Overcoming unhelpful thinking patterns'.

**EXAMPLES OF WORRIES OR LOOSE ENDS
AND HOW TO RESOLVE THEM**

Worry/loose ends		Steps to resolve	
1.	Argument with a friend or colleague.	1.	Send them a text (first thing tomorrow). Arrange to meet to discuss tomorrow.
2.	Lots to do tomorrow.	2.	Write a list of things I want to do during the day after breakfast. Prioritise what 'needs' to be done.
3.	House in a mess and visitors coming.	3.	Allocate half an hour to work on the house over the next few days. Delegate/ask others to help.

How to deal with frustration about not being able to sleep

If you become frustrated about not being able to fall asleep, and worry about the possible 'negative' consequences the next day, it is likely that you will inhibit sleep further by trying harder to fall asleep. So:

- Do not try too hard to fall asleep.
- Tell yourself that 'sleep will come when it is ready', and that 'relaxing in bed is almost as good as being asleep'.
- Try to keep your eyes open in the darkened room, and as they (naturally) try to close, tell yourself to resist closing them for another few seconds. This procedure 'tempts' sleep to take over.
- Visualise a pleasing scene, such as a place where you have felt peaceful and relaxed, possibly on a holiday. Also try to imagine what you can smell, hear, feel, taste and touch to make the experience as full as possible. You may find it helpful to have a think about a couple of examples that you can try out in the daytime so that you will be prepared to use this strategy at night.
- While visualising your pleasing scene, you may find it helpful to do some calming breathing exercises, which will help your body to relax further. Please see Chapter 10 for more information about breathing exercises that may be helpful.

7

Planning activity and rest

Developing a good balance between activity and rest is a key component in helping you to manage your fatigue more effectively. This chapter will first help you to construct your initial programme of planned activity and rest. It will then help you to work towards some of the targets that you have set for yourself in Chapter 7 by showing you how to gradually increase, change or add in new activities.

When can I plan my first activity programme?

You can plan your first activity programme as soon as you feel that you have a clear idea of your overall pattern of activity and rest in the day and your pattern of sleep at night. This will probably be about two weeks after starting to complete your diaries. The aim of your first activity programme will be to stabilise or make consistent what you are already doing rather than to make any big changes.

Different programmes for different circumstances

Because chronic fatigue affects people in such diverse ways, we have separated this chapter into two sections. Although you are likely to find one section more applicable to your own circumstances than the other, we would recommend that you read them both.

- *Section 1* aims to help people who have significantly cut down all or most of the things they used to do. (See page 105.)
- *Section 2* aims to help people who are able to manage certain aspects of their lives, such as work, studying or managing their home but are unable to do other activities such as see friends or exercise regularly. (Please turn to page 117.)

Section 1:
Planning activity and rest for people whose activities have greatly reduced

We have previously discussed factors that frequently contribute to the maintenance of chronic fatigue, such as a poor sleep pattern, too much rest or too little rest, etc. We hope that by now you will have identified some of the things that might be contributing to keeping your own fatigue going. Have another look at the vicious cycle of fatigue that you drew on page 35 as a reminder.

It is likely that you will probably have tried a variety of things to help you feel better, but you may feel that you are taking two steps forward and one step back.

A very common factor that contributes to the maintenance of chronic fatigue is reduced activity and increased rest. As we explained in Chapter 1, reduced activity and prolonged periods of rest may cause physical changes in the body. These changes cause unpleasant sensations and symptoms that can be very distressing and often lead people to have an erratic pattern of rest and activity, dependent on how they feel.

Your symptoms may be so severe that you spend much of your time confined to bed or the house, and your days and nights run into each other. You may find that *any* activity is exhausting: brushing your hair, talking, walking around a room, getting dressed or washed. On the other hand, you may feel a bit better on some days and that you can do a little more. However, as a result of 'doing too much' on the days when you feel a little better, you may become more fatigued and find that other symptoms increase, so that you cannot do very much on the following days.

Why does rest sometimes not feel restful?

We all need adequate rest and relaxation to be healthy. People with chronic fatigue often find that they rest more than they used to, but rarely find themselves more refreshed as a result. This may be for the following reasons:

- Your body does not get a chance to get used to a regular routine, as you may be resting in response to your symptoms of fatigue and pain, rather than in a planned way.
- Although you probably *feel* that you need more rest, too much rest can be counterproductive as it may lead to disturbed sleep and reduced physical fitness; in fact, it can make you feel *more* tired and lethargic.
- It may be difficult for you to relax properly, as you may find it hard to 'switch off' when you try to rest e.g. you may be thinking about all the jobs that you need to do, or you may be worrying about things you are not able to do.

In order to establish a better balance of activity and rest, it is helpful to plan in advance what you are going to do each day: this is what you will be doing in creating an 'activity programme'.

Things to consider when planning a programme of activity and rest

- The key to becoming more active is to aim for *consistency* and *regularity* in both activity and rest, in the first instance. It is important that you plan small chunks of activity at regular intervals, rather than long periods of occasional activity. As you increase your everyday activities you will gradually become stronger and be able to cut down on rest.

- Try to plan to do about the same amount of activity, and have the same number of rests, each day. This may be difficult for practical reasons, but aim for as much consistency as possible.

- When writing your first activity programme, aim for about as much 'overall' activity as you are having at present in a given week. So, for example, if you do all your cleaning on one day and it takes you two hours, break it down into four half-hourly chunks spread throughout the week.

- It is important to think about what you will do during your rest/relaxation time. Rests are a time for you to try to relax. What you do in your rest time will depend on your level of fatigue and the things that you find relaxing. Some people may find that reading is relaxing; for others, reading may be a major activity. Listening to audiobooks, music, radio programmes or watching television are other relaxing things you may consider. Some people like to relax with their partner, children or pet(s), watch the birds outside, paint or knit. The important thing is that the rest time is used as a break from activity.

- Try to avoid using your bed for resting or sleeping during the day, however tired you feel. Sleeping in the day or resting in your bedroom is likely to affect your sleep at night. However, as we mentioned in the previous chapter, if you live in one room – e.g. in a bedsit or student accommodation – and have nowhere else to relax, then cover your bed during the day so that it feels different when you get into bed at night.

Please refer to your 'target breakdown sheets' on pages 86–88 for guidance on some of the activities that you may like to include in your activity programme.

Steps to creating an activity programme

Planning activities

- Write a list of activities that you would like to do during the next week on your activity programme. Examples can be found on the next few pages and a blank activity programme for you to photocopy is provided on page 126).

- For each activity, specify how *often* you want to do it and how *long* you want to spend on it on each occasion: e.g. 'read for fifteen minutes every other day'; 'tidy up for half an hour every day'.
- Use your activity diaries for guidance on the *time* to be spent on each activity during the week to make sure you don't overdo it.
- Remember to make your activity times *manageable chunks*, rather than one long session: e.g. if you have been doing one solid hour of housework each day, divide it into three chunks of twenty minutes each.
- Remember to include strategies to improve your sleep such as getting up at a regular time in the morning.

Planning rests/relaxation

- Look at the activity diaries that you have completed and estimate the average amount of rest taken each day.
- Write down on your activity programme the *number* of rests to be taken each day, and the *length* of each rest.

You may like to use the formula below to calculate your initial amount of resting or relaxing.

- Look at your activity diaries and add up the total number of hours of rest that you have had during the period in which you completed them.

- Divide the number of hours of rest by the number of days you have completed your diaries: this will give you an estimate of the amount of rest to be taken each day.

Example 1: Total rest over 14 days = 42 hours.
42 ÷ 14 = 3
Amount of rest to be taken each day: 3 hours.
Example 2: Total rest over 7 days = 35 hours
35 ÷ 7 = 5
Amount of rest to be taken each day: 5 hours

Examples of an initial activity programme

For someone who is resting for about three hours a day:

- To get up and get dressed by 8 a.m.
- To have three one-hour rests in a chair (e.g. at 10 a.m., 2 p.m. and 6 p.m.) every day.
- To go for two fifteen-minute walks every day.
- To read for twenty minutes twice a day.
- To do chores for half an hour twice a day.
- To talk to friends on the phone/email/Facebook for fifteen minutes twice a day.
- To go to bed when sleepy at around 11.00 p.m.
- To meet a friend weekly locally for one hour.

For someone who is resting for about six hours a day:

- To get up and get dressed by 9.00 a.m.
- To go for two ten-minute walks every day.
- To do chores for fifteen minutes four times a day.
- To talk to friends on the phone/email/Facebook for ten minutes, three times a week.
- To read for ten minutes twice a day.
- To rest in a chair for six one-hour periods, evenly spaced throughout the day.
- To go to bed after 10.30 p.m. when sleepy.

For someone who is resting for most of the day:

- To get out of bed by 9.00 a.m.
- To rest for fifty minutes each hour.
- To do some activity (specify what) for ten minutes each hour, e.g. get washed and brush teeth by 9.30 a.m. every day; get dressed by 10.30 a.m. every day; read for ten minutes twice every day; wash and dry dishes twice a day; walk around for at least one minute per hour, prepare vegetables, wash hair, shower, do some admin, read or play with children.

Recording your activities

You will already be used to recording your activities in your activity diary. It can be helpful to continue to write down what you are doing for each hour of the day in your activity diary as you begin your activity programme. It will help you to keep track of your progress.

Remember though that these goals are only suggestions and you may not feel they are appropriate for you. They are meant to be examples of specific SMART goals, by which we mean that they should be *specific*, *measurable*, *achievable*, *realistic* and *timed*.

What to expect when you start your activity programme

As we mentioned in Chapter 3, your symptoms may increase slightly when you start your activity programme. However, this is usually temporary and occurs as a result of developing a new routine. Even though you may feel like resting more, try to persevere with your programme. In time, your body will get used to your new routine and gradually any temporary increased symptoms should subside.

Increasing your activity levels

Once you have established a more consistent pattern of activity and rest, you will be ready to increase – *gradually* – the amount of activity you do each day. This will probably be about two to four weeks after you start your initial activity programme. By this time, we hope that you will feel that you are managing your planned activities and planned rests more consistently.

- Look at your activity programme and ask yourself, for each different activity: 'How successful was I at completing it?'

For activities that you feel that you have achieved fairly easily and consistently, you may want to slightly increase the time you spend on the activity. Think about increasing the time by about 10 to 20 per cent. So, for example, if you have been walking for fifteen minutes, twice daily (total half an hour daily), you may increase your total walking time by three to six minutes to thirty-three to thirty-six minutes per day. If you have been doing emails/admin for ten minutes a day, you could add on another one or two minutes per day.

For activities that you feel you've only had a moderate amount of success with, you may want to give yourself another week or so on this activity and then try to build up in a week or so. It may also be useful to consider what stood in the way of your carrying out your goals/activity as consistently as you'd hoped. You can then put something in place to help you over the next week. So, for example, if you haven't managed to get up at the time you had planned, you could turn up the volume of your alarm or move your alarm to the other side of the room so that you have to get out of bed.

For activities that you have not achieved, you may wish to consider whether you had set your target level too high and reduce it slightly. On the other hand, you may feel that you have had a difficult week for a number of reasons and decide to repeat the activity next week. If this is the case, think about steps to help you achieve your target.

How often should I review and make changes to my activity programme?

We would recommend that you set aside fifteen to twenty minutes each week to review your activity programme. This will give you the opportunity to assess your progress and help you to decide whether you can make any changes to your activity programme for the next week.

When should I introduce new activities?

- It is sometimes hard to know when to introduce new activities. *Consider introducing things when you feel that you are managing your programme reasonably well.* This may be a few weeks after starting your activity programme. Introducing new activities too soon, though, can backfire, so try to do things at a steady pace as opposed to a gallop.
- When you have achieved one of your targets, you may find that you have the time to introduce another activity. So, for example, if you have achieved a target of going out socially once a week, you may feel like

adding a new social activity each week or perhaps doing something different, such as a regular exercise class or evening class.

- Sometimes you will find that you plan targets that are not manageable for a variety of reasons. So, for example, if one of your targets was to go swimming each week and the pool was closed for cleaning, you might substitute another exercise for swimming. If you planned to send emails for fifteen minutes three times a week and your computer breaks down, perhaps write to friends instead.

- Once you reduce your resting time, you will be able to include another activity or increase one that you are already doing. So, for example, if you have successfully reduced your rest from one hour to thirty minutes, you could use this extra time to include another activity.

It is not necessary for your fatigue to have decreased for you to increase or start a new activity.

How do I decrease my rests?

Gradually cut down the *amount* of time you spend resting at first. So, for example, if you rest for an hour three times a day, you may start by reducing each rest by ten minutes. Or, if you rest for half an hour six times a day, you may want to reduce three of the rests by five minutes and leave the others at half an hour.

If you have a lot of rest periods in the day, you may want to reduce the *number* of rests you take.

It is important that you continue to include some short rests in the day, even if you are feeling better; otherwise you may get into the cycle of pushing yourself too hard for too long and having to take long 'recovery' rests. We recommend that you have at least a mid-morning and a mid-afternoon break, as well as one at lunchtime.

Section 2:
Planning activity and rest for people who can maintain an area of life such as work or study but do little else

In Chapter 3, we discussed factors that frequently contribute to the maintenance of chronic fatigue. We hope that by now you will have identified some of the things that you feel may be responsible for keeping your own fatigue going. Have another look at the vicious cycle of fatigue that you drew on page 35 as a reminder.

You may find that you are able to 'keep going' at work, manage your home or study for long periods, but that in the evenings and at weekends you spend most of your time resting or sleeping in an attempt to recover for the following week. This pattern can be very frustrating, causing you to miss out on pleasurable activities such as seeing friends or family, taking days out, doing some exercise, or pursuing your hobbies.

The key to feeling better is to try to make your life as balanced as possible. It is therefore important that you identify areas that you could change. For example, do you find that you tend to keep going at work without taking breaks? Do you find that you do not sit down at home until you have taken your children to school, tidied the house and done the shopping? Do you find that you do not leave work until you have completed everything there is to do, even if it is late? Do you study for hours without taking a break and then have to sleep for a couple of days because you feel so fatigued? Do you feel that you have too many responsibilities? Are you trying to study as well as work full time? If the answer to some of the above questions is yes, then maybe you could consider some of the following ideas.

- Could you leave work a little earlier?
- Could you have a proper lunch-break, instead of eating a sandwich at your desk?
- Could you postpone the cleaning, washing, preparing meals and so on, and sit down for half an hour?
- Could you consider getting a cleaner/gardener for a few hours?
- Could you plan one or two pleasurable activities each week?
- Could you put aside one hour for yourself each day?
- Could you break up your studies with a brisk walk?
- Could you ask others at home to take on more of the chores or share the cooking?
- Could you get a later deadline to complete your coursework?

It is important to plan in advance what you are going to do each day by creating an activity programme. This will help you to balance your time between things that you have to do – for example work, studying, or managing your home

– with pleasurable activities such as seeing friends and having time to relax.

Things to consider when planning a programme of activity and rest/relaxation

- Try to include a few short breaks each day in your busy schedule. Even if you are working in a demanding job or looking after young children, it should be possible to ensure that you have *at least* a fifteen-minute break in the morning and afternoon, as well as a lunch-break of at least half an hour.
- Do *not* be tempted to carry out long periods of activities without breaks, even if you feel that you have a lot of energy. You are likely to pay for it later and *feel* that you need to rest, leading you to miss out on other things you want to do.
- Try *not* to be tempted to catch up with rest at the weekend. However, it's absolutely fine to ensure that you have time to relax. Once you start taking regular breaks in the day, you will hopefully feel less fatigued at the weekend and have a bit more energy.
- Refer to your target breakdown sheet on pages 86–8 for guidance on some of the activities that you may like to include in your activity programme.
- Try to plan a few 'pleasurable' activities for the weekend, as well as a bit of time to catch up with chores.

Steps to creating an activity programme

Planning activities

- Write a list of activities that you would like to do during the next week on your activity programme. (A blank activity diary can be found on page 126 for you to photocopy if you wish.) For each activity, specify how *often* you want to do it and how *long* you want to spend on it on each occasion: e.g. 'Leave work by 5 p.m. two days a week'; 'Meet a friend once a week for one hour'; 'Have a daily half-hour lunch-break away from my desk.'

- When writing your first activity programme, aim for about as much 'overall' activity as you are having at present. So, for example, if you do all of your chores on one day, break up the amount of time that you usually spend on them into small chunks to do on two or three days.

- Remember to make your activity times *manageable chunks*, rather than one long session: e.g. if you plan to do some gardening at a weekend, plan two half-hour periods rather than a solid hour.

Planning relaxation time

Whether you are working, studying or managing a home and/or looking after children, regular time for relaxation is important. Taking regular breaks can help you to feel a lot better and give you more energy to do the things that you want to do in the evenings and at weekends. What you find relaxing is a very personal thing. It may be reading a book, listening to music, doing a puzzle, watching a film or taking a long bath.

In order to plan relaxation time:

- Look at the activity diaries and add up the total amount of rest/relaxation that you have had during the period you completed them: e.g., if you have completed your diaries for fourteen days then add up the amount of rest you took for those days. (You may find that on some days you rested very little, but at weekends you rested for much of the time.)
- Divide the total amount of rest/breaks you have taken during the past fourteen days (or number of days you have completed them) to calculate the approximate amount of relaxation time to be taken each day. (This will mean increasing rests on some days and reducing rest on others.)

Example:
Total rest over 14 days = 28 hours
$28 \div 14 = 2$ hours
Amount of rest/relaxation to be taken each day = 2 hours

- Write down on your activity programme the number of breaks/rests to be taken each day, and the length of each one. If you are working or studying, you will need to consider what is achievable in relation to your commitments. For example, you might take two fifteen-minute breaks and a single one-hour break each day; or you might take three half-hour breaks each day.

- Think about how your weekend differs to the week-days when you may be working. Think about doing enjoyable activities on your days off as well as chores.

Examples of an initial activity programme

For someone who is working:

- To have at least two fifteen-minute breaks and a half-hour lunch-break every day.
- To leave work on time at least twice a week.
- To walk for half an hour five days a week.
- To spend one hour daily doing something relaxing e.g. listening to music, watching television.
- To go out socially once a week for two hours.
- To go to bed around 11.00 p.m. every day during the week.

For someone who cares for family/home all of the time:

- To have one fifteen-minute break at home in the morning and one in the afternoon every day.
- To have a half-hour break at lunchtime every day.

- To spend one hour, twice a day, cleaning/cooking/ doing other chores.
- To go for two fifteen-minute walks every day.
- To go out with friends and/or partner every week for two hours.
- To stop chores by 9.00 p.m. every day.
- To spend at least one hour a day on a hobby or reading.

For someone studying at college or university:

- To get up by 9:00 a.m. daily.
- To study for two hours each day.
- To walk for twenty minutes daily.
- To attend all my lectures.
- To prepare one fresh meal each day.
- To meet a friend twice weekly for one and half hours.
- To switch off my computer/phone by 10:00 p.m. daily.
- To relax every afternoon for one hour.

Recording your activities

You will already be used to recording your activities in your activity diary. It can be helpful to continue to write down details of what you are doing in your activity diary once you have begun your activity programme so that you can keep track of your progress.

What to expect when you start your activity programme

This will depend on the sort of activity programme that you have set for yourself. If the main focus of your programme has been to introduce some regular planned time for relaxation, leave work earlier, ask other people to help you with chores, etc., you may find that you feel a little less fatigued. On the other hand, if you have changed your routine quite a lot with, for example, shorter more frequent breaks, a regular getting-up time, even at the weekend, more regular exercise rather than short bursts of longer exercise, you may notice a slight increase in your fatigue for a few weeks or so.

If you notice a slight increase in your symptoms, do try to maintain your activity programme as far as possible. Your symptoms should gradually decrease after a few weeks.

Changing your activity levels or introducing new activities

- *Once you have established a more consistent pattern of activity and rest* throughout the week and feel that you are managing your activity programme reasonably well, you will be in a position to *gradually* introduce new activities or change your programme in some way. So, for example, you might decide to build in a hobby or social event that you have identified as a target. This may be between two and four weeks after you start your programme.

- When you have achieved a particular target, you may find that you have the time to introduce another activity, e.g. if you have completed a course at college, you may plan to do another. Or, if you have achieved a target of leaving work on time twice a week, you may consider leaving work on time every day. Alternatively, you may choose to start working on a new target e.g. meeting up with friends twice a week.

- Sometimes you will find that you plan targets that are not manageable for a variety of reasons. So, for example, if one of your targets was to go to a yoga class once a week, but the class was cancelled because not enough people enrolled, then you may decide to join a Pilates class or practise yoga exercises at home until the class reopens.

- It is *not* necessary for your fatigue to have decreased for you to increase or start a new activity.

How often should I review my programme?

- Reviewing your programme each week will help you to assess your progress, even though you may make changes to it only, say, once a fortnight, or once a month. From now on, set aside fifteen to twenty minutes a week to review your homework and to plan your next activity programme.

- Remember to make time for relaxation, with no specific activity allocated.

ACTIVITY PROGRAMME

1. _____
2. _____
3. _____
4. _____
5. _____
6. _____
7. _____
8. _____
9. _____
10. _____
11. _____
12. _____
13. _____
14. _____
15. _____
16. _____
17. _____
18. _____
19. _____
20. _____

FOR EVERYONE!

Keeping a target achievement record

When you feel that you have established a good routine and

are *consistently* managing your activity programme, you may feel that your activity and sleep diaries are no longer necessary and decide to stop using them. However, you may find it helpful to continue to track your progress by keeping a target achievement record instead. This record will help you track your progress and requires you to make a tick in a box, rather than actually writing details of what you have done.

An example of a completed target achievement record, and a blank record sheet for you to photocopy, are included on pages 128–9.

What do I have to do?

- Write down the contents of your activity programme on the left-hand side of your target achievement record: e.g. get up by 8 a.m., read a newspaper for fifteen minutes daily, etc.
- Tick the appropriate boxes as you complete these activities throughout the day, so that you can easily monitor your progress.
- For targets that you do not attempt or achieve, put an X in the appropriate box or leave it blank.
- For targets that you attempt, but do not manage to carry on for the planned time, record how long you did manage: e.g. against 'Go for a half-hour walk' you might note '20 minutes'.
- If you start using the target achievement records and find after a week or so that you do not like them or find them helpful, then you can always return to using activity diaries.

Sample completed target achievement record

Fortnight beginning ....

Target	Mon	Tue	Wed	Thu	Fri	Sat	Sun	Mon	Tue	Wed	Thu	Fri	Sat	Sun
To get up by 8 a.m.	✓	8.20	✓	✓	✓	9.00	8.45	✓	✓	✓	✓	8.15	9.30	9.10
To walk for half an hour twice daily	✓X	✓✓	20 mins	✓✓	✓✓	✓X	X✓	✓✓	✓✓	15 mins	✓✓	✓✓	X 45 mins	✓✓
To read for half an hour twice daily	✓✓	✓✓	X✓	✓✓	✓✓	X	✓X	✓✓	✓✓	✓✓	✓✓	40 mins	XX	✓✓
To have an hour's rest in chair at 10 a.m.	✓	✓	✓	✓	½ hrs	1¼ hrs	✓	✓	✓	✓	✓	45 mins	X	✓
To do chores for half an hour twice daily	✓✓	✓	✓X	✓✓	✓✓	10 mins	✓X	✓✓	✓✓	✓✓	✓✓	✓✓	XX	X✓
To have an hour's rest in chair at 1 p.m.	✓	✓	1¼ hrs	✓	✓	2 hrs	✓	✓	✓	✓	½ hrs	✓	✓	✓
To meet a friend for coffee twice weekly for 1 hr		✓			✓			✓			met for lunch			
To swim twice weekly for 20 mins			✓			✓			✓	✓				✓
To have an hour's rest in chair at 4 p.m.	✓	✓	✓	✓	✓	✓	✓	✓	✓	✓	1½ hrs	45 mins	X	✓
To prepare evening meal three times weekly for family	✓			✓		✓			✓	✓		✓	✓	✓
Enquire about voluntary work		✓ online												
Comments					late night	felt v. ill	better day			enjoyed swim				

128

Target achievement record

Fortnight beginning ....

Target	Mon	Tue	Wed	Thu	Fri	Sat	Sun	Mon	Tue	Wed	Thu	Fri	Sat	Sun

8

Symptom management

In this chapter, we offer one way to help you deal with unpleasant symptoms you may be experiencing. In the first chapter, we talked about common symptoms reported by people with chronic fatigue syndrome, including fatigue, pain, dizziness, and sensitivity to light and noise, and summarised some of the physiology behind them. Whatever symptoms you are experiencing, they are likely to fluctuate in intensity and may at times be both distressing and debilitating.

When experiencing unpleasant symptoms, it can be difficult not to focus on them. You may find that your attention is constantly brought back to them and that you notice when they get better or worse. You may find that you focus more on your body than you would like. This attentional process is difficult to control. However, focusing your attention on symptoms, however natural and automatic it seems, can have negative consequences. Not only can it intensify them, but it can also increase your awareness of normal bodily sensations such as your heart rate, breathing, temperature, etc. Any concerns or worries about your health that you have may intensify.

Although many of the behavioural strategies in the book may lead to symptoms reducing, it may be helpful to have another way of addressing symptoms more directly.

Attention training

Attentional training was originally developed to enable individuals to shift the focus of their attention away from worry. It has subsequently been used to help people successfully shift their attention away from unpleasant symptoms or bodily sensations. We outline below a task-focusing exercise to help you with this.

Task focusing

When you are doing tasks such as washing up, cooking, cleaning your teeth, tidying a drawer, dusting, etc., you may be aware of lots of different things. For instance, you may be aware of thoughts going through your mind; some of these thoughts may be about the next task or general thoughts about the day, but some may be to do with how you are feeling, e.g. feeling fatigued, having sore muscles that are making the activity difficult. Learning to focus on the task in hand provides a great opportunity for you to practise training your attention towards whatever you are doing, therefore leading to less focus on your thoughts and bodily sensations.

What do I have to do?

- First of all, write a list in the space provided below of at least five tasks that you would like to practise focusing your attention on.

Task 1 . . . .

Task 2 . . . .

Task 3 . . . .

Task 4 . . . .

Task 5 . . . .

- Choose one of the above tasks to try out your first task focusing exercise. You may find it helpful to start on the least complicated one. So, brushing your teeth or ironing may be more straightforward than cooking.
- Plan *when* you are going to do your task focusing exercise and add this target to your activity programme.
- You may like to try one task focusing exercise per day for the first week to see how you get on. You can then gradually build up the number that you do over the coming weeks.
- During your task focusing exercise, we would like you to bring your attention to your senses of sight, smell, touch, taste and sound.

    Sight: What can you actually see? What colours do

you notice? What are the surfaces like? Are there cracks/crevices/different shades of colour?

Smell: What can you smell? Are there any smells? Different ones?

Touch: What do the things that you are doing in your task feel like? Do you feel different textures? Are they rough or smooth? What temperatures can you feel? Hot or cold?

Taste: What can you taste? Is there more than one flavour? Does the flavour change in different parts of your mouth?

Sound: What can you hear? Are the sounds associated with your task or in another part of the room or outside? How many sounds do you notice?

- Complete the task-focusing exercise form on page 135, which has been left blank for you to photocopy.

  ° Write on the form the task that you have chosen.
  ° Write down what you noticed (sight/smell, etc).
  ° Give yourself a rating of how much attention was focused on 'yourself', e.g. awareness of bodily sensations/symptoms or thoughts/worries. In the same column, rate how much you were focused on the 'task'.
  ° Note any comments in the comments column.

Please see overleaf for an example of a completed task focusing exercise form.

Task focusing exercise

Date	Task	What did I notice?	Where was my attention focused?	Comments
	Brushing teeth	**Sight**: two-tone blue toothbrush, gleaming white toothpaste **Smell**: sweet and minty **Touch**: bristly feeling on my gums **Taste**: minty **Sound**: rhythmic sound of toothbrush, tap running, radio on in background	Self: 40 per cent Task: 60 per cent	Did better than I thought I would! However, noticed thoughts about going to the dentist as I haven't been for ages.

Task focusing exercise

Date	Task	What did I notice?	Where was my attention focused?	Comments

Task focusing exercise

After you have completed the task focusing exercise a few times and have had some success with noticing what you can see, hear, taste, etc., you can experiment with going into the task with an 'open mind', by which we mean not specifically focussing on your senses. If you then find that your attention starts to be drawn to your symptoms or worrying thoughts, etc., you can focus on what you can see, hear, taste, etc again.

Also, you can build up the number of things each day that you try to focus on in the way described in the task focusing. Examples may include the following:

- Going for a walk.
- Brushing the cat.
- Having a bath.
- Stroking your pet.
- Swimming.
- On the bus or train.

Points to bear in mind

- Task focusing can take a while to master; therefore don't give up!
- Use the task focusing exercise record as long as you find it to be useful.
- If you find yourself distracted during your tasks, then maybe choose a shorter more straightforward one. We often advise people to start with brushing their teeth.

9

Overcoming unhelpful thinking patterns

This chapter aims to help you to deal with unhelpful or troubling thoughts. If you have read Chapter 8 on symptom management, you may have tried the task focusing exercises and hopefully had some success in reducing symptoms and associated worries.

This chapter helps you to deal with worries and unhelpful thoughts in a different way. First, it aims to help you to understand a little more about how the way we think about things can affect us. It then describes strategies to help you to 'challenge' unhelpful thought patterns that may be making life more difficult for you.

We have divided this chapter into three sections:

Section 1: Understanding how our thinking affects us

Section 2: Tackling unhelpful thoughts

Section 3: Tackling unhelpful assumptions and negative core beliefs

Section 1:
Understanding how our thinking affects us

In this section, we discuss the relationship between our thoughts, feelings, behaviours and physical reactions, in which we include normal bodily sensations such as feeling hot and cold as well as fatigue, pain, etc. We then specifically focus on helping you to further understand how the way we *think* about things may affect us.

Our lives are influenced by five interconnected areas:

- thoughts (beliefs, images, memories);
- feelings (moods or emotions);
- behaviours (what we do: e.g. activity, sleep, rest);
- physical reactions (fatigue, pain, sensitivity to light and noise, dizziness, changes in energy levels, sleep, appetite, etc.);
- environment (what happens in our life, both past and present).

Please see the diagram on the next page to see how each area directly influences the other four areas.

ENVIRONMENT/LIFE CHANGES/SITUATIONS

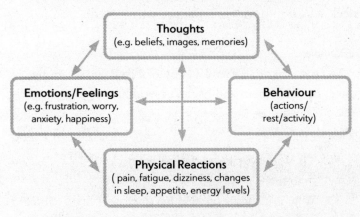

Figure 9.1 How aspects of our lives interconnect

For example:

- If a friend who you haven't heard from for a while sends you a message (behaviour), you may think, 'It's so nice to hear from him' (thought) and feel happy (emotion).
- If you fall over and graze your knee (behaviour), it is likely that you would have pain (physical reaction) and, depending on how bad the cut is, you may feel dizzy or sick (physical reactions) and feel annoyed (emotion) with yourself for not looking where you were going.
- If it's a warm and sunny day (environment) following a few grey days, you may think 'At last! I'm so pleased it's sunny today' (thoughts) and be happy (emotion) and may go out for a walk/sit in the park (behaviour).

You could look at the above examples and interpret them in a different way. That is because there are a number of ways of thinking about any situation. The way that you think about the situation is likely to determine how you feel, which in turn will influence what you do.

Example:
You sent a text to a friend a couple of days ago to arrange to meet up with them and haven't heard back.

Possible thoughts	*Possible feelings*
• They always take a while to get back to me.	*Content*
• Why is it always me that has to chase people up?	*Irritated*
• They clearly aren't bothered about seeing me.	*Upset*
• What have I done wrong?	
• _____	_____
• _____	_____

You can see from the example above that there are a variety of ways of looking at the situation. You may look at it in a different way; there is space for you to add your own thought and feeling.

Each different thought leads to a different feeling or emotion: e.g. contentment, irritation, upset. It is likely that these thoughts and feelings lead people to behave in different ways. For example:

• The 'content' person may send a further brief text to their friend to check that they had received it or wait to hear from them in a relaxed manner.

- The 'irritated' person may be a bit 'off hand' with their friend if/when they hear from them again.
- The 'upset' person may continue to feel sad and spend time thinking about what they have done wrong.

What would the example that you have written lead you to do?

- _____

_____

At times, it can be advantageous to change the way we *think* about things. If we change the way we *think* about something it can then change what we do (behaviour) and lead to positive changes in the way we feel (emotions) and our physical reactions. So, using the example above, if the 'upset' person changed their thoughts to 'They often take a while to get back to me', they are likely to feel 'happier' and be able to get on with their day in a more relaxed manner.

Changes in our life will influence our emotions, physical feelings, thoughts and behaviour. It is likely that promotion, passing exams, winning the Lottery, a new positive relationship and so on will make us feel happy, feel good about ourselves, and inclined to celebrate. Failing exams, illness, relationship break-ups, family difficulties, bereavements and financial problems are changes in our lives that may make us feel upset, worried, stressed and tired, and may lead us to feel down, withdraw from others, and so on. The way we think about things may also be influenced by past experiences; we shall look at this in a bit more depth in Section 3.

Section 2:
Tackling unhelpful thoughts

It is perfectly normal to have unhelpful thoughts from time to time – we all do! However, if you are suffering from chronic fatigue syndrome or in fact any illness that is making you fatigued, it may be difficult to remain positive. This is understandable when you feel unwell, your life has become restricted and your future appears uncertain. You may have experienced a lack of understanding from family, friends or health professionals about your health problems, which may have contributed to you feeling demoralised or a little alone. You may feel frustrated about the things you are not able to do at the moment and worry about your health. These negative thoughts and feelings can make it harder for you to make progress in overcoming your illness. This section offers some ways to tackle these thoughts in order to help you to feel less distressed in general and to be able to move forward in a more confident and positive way.

As we mentioned at the beginning of the chapter, at times, you may feel that you are having difficulty with making progress with your programme. You may have thoughts such as:

- My progress seems very slow.
- I haven't managed much of my activity programme, it's just too hard!

142

- Getting up at the same time each day is unrealistic!
- I seem to be taking two steps forward and one step back.

These are examples of 'unhelpful thoughts' that may make it difficult at times for you to continue with your activity programme.

We have noticed that many people with CFS have unhelpful thoughts that can be divided into two main areas:

- Fears or worries about their illness.
- High personal standards and self-expectations.

Fears or worries about the illness

Here is an example of how an unhelpful thought related to fears about illness affected other areas of a person's life:

Situation	*Woke up feeling exhausted and very achy after walking too far the previous day.*
Thought	*I've clearly overdone it!*
Behaviour	*Rested for most of the day.*
Emotions	*Worried about making fatigue worse.*
	Annoyed for giving in to tiredness.
Physical reaction	*Increase in physical symptoms e.g. fatigue and aching muscles.*

Can you think of any personal examples of how thoughts about your fatigue have influenced other aspects of your life? If so, please write them in the spaces provided below.

Situation _____

_____

Thought _____

_____

Behaviour _____

_____

Emotion _____

_____

Physical reaction _____

Having extremely high personal standards and self-expectations

Many people with CFS say that before they developed their illness they were very busy, energetic people: driven, conscientious with high expectations of themselves and sometimes others. They would sometimes describe them-selves as perfectionists.

What is perfectionism?

Perfectionism is a concept that doesn't fit reality, as what one person sees as 'perfect' may not be considered 'perfect' by another person. Let's take the example of eating a meal in a restaurant or at a reception where there are other people eating the same food, or even sitting round the table at home. One person may comment on the food being perfect, but others may comment that it's a bit cold/underdone/bland/rich, etc. Although there's no specific definition, we understand that perfectionism involves the following:

- Relentless striving for extremely high standards (for yourself and/or others).
- Judging your self-worth based mostly on your ability to strive for and achieve such unrelenting standards.
- Experiencing negative consequences of setting such unrelenting standards, yet trying to maintain them despite the cost to you.

You may find that your fatigue has made it very difficult to maintain previous high standards or to do as much as you used to, and this can lead to:

- being overly self-critical;
- worrying about starting new things, fearing not being able to complete them or do them well enough;
- doubting your judgement; making it harder to complete tasks;

- focusing on the things that you *haven't* done;
- feeling guilty about relaxing if you haven't completed a task to your satisfaction;
- feeling frustrated about doing so much less than you used to be able to do.

Here is an example of how unhelpful thoughts relating to perfectionism affected Sarah.

Situation	*Didn't study for as long as I had planned.*
Thought	*I should have handed in the essay by now.*
	I've missed another deadline.
Emotions	'Frustrated' *about not completing the task.* 'Worried' *about missing deadline.*
Behaviour	*Unable to relax or concentrate on any one thing.*
Physical reaction	*Feeling more fatigued.*

Can you think of any personal examples of how 'perfectionist' thoughts have influenced other aspects of your life since you developed fatigue? If so, please write them in the spaces provided below.

Situation _____

_____

Thought _____

_____

Behaviour _____

_____

Emotion _____

_____

Physical reaction _____

As well as the unhelpful thoughts mentioned above, you may from time to time have unhelpful thoughts about a variety of things related or unrelated to your fatigue: for example, relationship issues, work, finances, friendship or family issues. These thoughts may also make you feel a bit upset or low in mood and may, in turn, negatively affect your fatigue.

Characteristics of unhelpful thoughts

Unhelpful thoughts are:

- *automatic:* as with all thoughts, unhelpful ones tend to pop into our head rapidly and unexpectedly, without any deliberate or conscious effort;
- *distorted:* they are usually not entirely accurate;
- *plausible:* we accept them as facts, and do not question them;
- *persistent:* they can be difficult to switch off;
- *durable:* it can be useful to view unhelpful thoughts as prejudices, as they can be hard to change.

How do I identify and record my unhelpful thoughts?

Over the next week or so, try to notice what goes through your mind when you have a strong feeling, a strong reaction to something, a worsening of symptoms or a change in your mood.

Write down your 'unhelpful' thoughts as soon as possible so that you remember them in detail. You may like to use the headings shown in the 'unhelpful thoughts diary' on the next page. You can either photocopy the blank diary that can be found on page 152, or use your phone, diary or whatever suits you. However, try to use the headings as suggested on the form.

- In the 'Situation' column, write down what you were doing or thinking about just before having a strong feeling or change in your emotion/mood: e.g. thinking about the day ahead, meeting people you haven't seen for a while, arriving home after a busy day.
- In the 'Emotion' column, write down the feeling that you had just before or at the time you had the unhelpful thought(s). Then write down the intensity of your emotion on a 0–100 per cent scale. If you find that a percentage scale does not work for you, then rate your emotion using words such as 'mild', 'moderate' or 'severe'.
- In the 'Unhelpful thoughts' column, write down the actual thought that went through your mind. If you have more than one unhelpful thought connected with the situation, then write them all down.

Unhelpful thoughts diary

Date	Situation	Emotion	Unhelpful thoughts
	What was I doing at the time of the thoughts?	How did I feel? Rate intensity of feeling (0–100%)	What thoughts went through my mind just before I started to feel this way? Rate belief in each thought (0–100%)

- Underneath, in the same column, write down how much you believe each thought, on a 0–100 per cent scale, where 0 per cent means that you do not believe it at all and 100 per cent means that you believe the thought completely, without any doubts.

Initially it can be difficult to detect your 'unhelpful' thoughts. After all, we are not used to focusing on what we are thinking about! However, with a bit of practice, it will become easier. Also, people sometimes feel a bit uncertain about writing down their unhelpful thoughts, as they may feel embarrassed about them or feel that they are rather trivial. However, it is important to acknowledge that this is the first step in overcoming your unhelpful thoughts, and if they are making you feel uncomfortable/worried/upset in some way, then they are not trivial!

An example of a completed unhelpful thoughts diary may be found on the next page.

For how long should I complete my unhelpful thoughts diary?

It is a good idea to write down your unhelpful thoughts for a few days, as it will give you a range of slightly different thoughts. Also, it can take a while to clearly distinguish between a *thought* and a *feeling* (emotion).

Example of a completed unhelpful thoughts diary

Date	Situation What was I doing at the time of the thoughts?	Emotion How did I feel? Rate intensity of feeling (0–100%)	Unhelpful thoughts What thoughts went through my mind just before I started to feel this way? Rate belief in each thought (0–100%)
1 Feb.	Trying to work on a piece for college.	Frustrated 70 per cent. Worried 60 per cent.	I just can't concentrate, I'll never get the work done in time.
3 Feb.	Meeting up with old friends from work.	Sad 80 per cent.	I feel so out of touch with everyone. I haven't worked for over a year and have nothing to contribute to the conversation. They must think that I am very boring.

Unhelpful thoughts diary

Date	Situation What was I doing at the time of the thoughts?	Emotion How did I feel? Rate intensity of feeling (0–100%)	Unhelpful thoughts What thoughts went through my mind just before I started to feel this way? Rate belief in each thought (0–100%)

Standing back from your unhelpful thoughts

Once you have identified any unhelpful thoughts, the very act of taking a step back from them can in itself be incredibly powerful, enabling you to see them for what they really are: *not* facts, just thoughts! It can also be helpful to prefix an unhelpful thought with 'I am having the thought that . . .' to help you to see that they are just thoughts.

So, for example:

- 'I'll never get that work assignment finished in time' becomes: *I am having the thought that I'll never get that work assignment finished in time.*
- 'I'm bound to feel exhausted if I meet my friends for a meal later' becomes: *I am having the thought that I'm bound to feel exhausted if I meet my friends for a meal later.*
- In the space below, write down an example of one of your unhelpful thoughts and at the front if it, add '*I'm having the thought that . . .*' What do you notice?

_____

_____

_____

Challenging unhelpful thoughts

Although some people find that standing back from their unhelpful thoughts can lead to a positive change in the way they feel, this is not always the case. This section shows you a couple of ways to challenge your thoughts, first by dissecting them and looking for 'thinking errors', and second by asking yourself a number of questions that will help you to look at your unhelpful thoughts in a more balanced way.

Why is it important to challenge unhelpful thoughts?

We have already discussed how the way we *think* about something will determine how we *feel*, and how the way we *feel* will often determine what we *do*. We have shown examples of this on page 144. You may have also written your own examples. Challenging these unhelpful thoughts is likely to help you to look at things in a more balanced way. This is likely to directly benefit how you feel and may influence what you choose to do.

When you start to challenge your unhelpful thoughts, we suggest that you look back at the unhelpful thoughts diaries that you have completed and pick just one thought that you would like to challenge, following the steps on the next few pages. When you have managed to challenge one unhelpful thought, you can either challenge another that you have already written down on your unhelpful thoughts diary or wait until you have another unhelpful thought and then challenge that one.

The 'new thoughts diary' expands on the unhelpful thoughts diary, adding four new stages:

1. *Evaluate your thoughts* to look for unhelpful thinking patterns.
2. *Answer questions* to consider evidence for and against your unhelpful thoughts.

3. *Suggest alternative thoughts* that are more realistic or helpful.

4. *Think of an action plan* to provide yourself with practical strategies to help you to break old habits of thinking and strengthen new ones.

Completing a new thoughts diary on this model will help you to monitor your progress in challenging your unhelpful thoughts. We have included two types of new thoughts diary for your use. The first one is more detailed than the second and some people prefer to use it to begin with; then, when they feel more confident with challenging their unhelpful thoughts, they move on to the second one. Detailed instructions on how to fill in both diaries, examples of completed diaries and blank diaries for you to photocopy can be found on pages 164–81.

When you start to challenge your unhelpful thoughts using your new thoughts diary, you can stop completing your unhelpful thoughts diary.

Step 1: Evaluate your unhelpful thoughts

Evaluating your thoughts involves detecting *thinking errors*: these are unhelpful thinking patterns that seem plausible, but often involve distortions of reality. This process will help you to stand back and dissect your thoughts rather than accepting them as facts.

- Look at the examples of unhelpful thinking patterns below.
- Look back at some of the unhelpful thoughts that you have written down. Can you identify any thinking errors?

You may notice that more than one thinking error applies to each thought and that you have a tendency towards one or two thinking errors in particular. This can be useful, as once you notice that you are making a particular thinking error repeatedly, it can immediately help you to take a step back from your thought and feel a bit better about your situation.

When you feel more confident about detecting thinking errors, you are ready to move on to the next step.

Unhelpful patterns of thinking

Unhelpful thinking pattern (thinking error/distortion)	Description	Example
All-or-nothing thinking, also called black-and-white thinking.	Looking at a situation as two extremes only, instead of a continuum.	'If I can't stay out until late, then there is no point in going out at all.'
Over-generalisation	Making a negative assumption that because something has happened once, it will happen again.	'I felt worse when I walked further last week, so I am bound to feel worse next time I walk further.'

Eliminating the positive	Dwelling on bad experiences and discounting positive aspects.	'I have had a terrible week and I have achieved nothing.'
'Should' and 'must' statements	Fixed expectations of how you think you or others should behave. You may overestimate how bad it is if these expect-ations are not met.	'I should be able to cope better by now; I'm not trying hard enough.' 'I must try harder!
Catastrophising	Getting things out of proportion, so that they appear worse than they really are.	'My muscles ache and I feel more tired today. I must be doing some permanent damage to myself.'
Emotional reasoning	Taking a feeling as being evidence of fact. You 'feel' (believe) it so strongly that you discount evidence to the contrary.	'I feel a real failure; I am no better now than I was a few months ago.'
Labelling	Putting a 'fixed' or 'global' label on yourself or others without considering evidence that doesn't support it.	'I'm incompetent.' 'My colleagues are totally insensitive.'
Mental filter	Paying undue attention to one negative detail instead of seeing the whole picture.	'One or two of my exam marks were dreadful (even though others were good); I don't deserve to pass my degree.'

Mind-reading	Believing that you know what others are thinking, without considering other possibilities.	'They think that just because I don't look ill, I am not ill.'
Personalisation	Blaming yourself or taking responsibility for something that wasn't entirely your fault.	'My doctor was irritable because I have seen him for a lot of appointments recently.'
Tunnel vision	Seeing only the negative aspects of a situation.	'I feel just as tired as I did three months ago; there has been no improvement in my illness.'
Predicting the future. Also called fortune-telling.	Making a negative assumption about the future.	'I'm bound to feel worse if I visit a friend tomorrow.'

Step 2: Finding alternative thoughts that are more helpful and realistic

This step involves you asking yourself questions to help you to look for more helpful and realistic alternatives to your unhelpful thoughts by:

- looking at the situation from another point of view;
- finding evidence that does not support them.

You may find some questions more helpful and relevant than others.

Choose one unhelpful thought and go through questions 1 to 10 with it. Write your answers down.

1. Have there been times in the past when I have had experiences that indicate that this thought is not true all of the time?
2. What might someone else think in this situation?
3. If my best friend or someone I loved had been in a similar situation, would I say the things that I have said to myself to him or to her? Yes or no? If no, what might I say to them?
4. If my best friend or someone who is close to me knew that I was thinking these things, what would they say to me?
5. What is the actual evidence or fact(s) that make this thought true?
6. Are there any small details or evidence that prove that this thought is wrong or not entirely accurate?
7. Am I blaming myself for something that wasn't entirely my fault?
8. Am I being too self-critical and expecting too much of myself?
9. What are the advantages of thinking this way?
10. What are the disadvantages of thinking this way?

After writing down your answers to the above questions, consider alternative thoughts. These should be more balanced and helpful than those that you have written in the 'Unhelpful thoughts' column of your unhelpful thoughts diary. One or two of your alternative thoughts may be the same as answers that you have written to questions 1 to 10.

Step 3: Writing an action plan

Detecting thinking errors and suggesting alternative thoughts may not always be enough to help you to feel better or to convince you that your thoughts are distorted or incorrect. Writing an action plan will provide you with practical strategies to help you to break old habits of thinking and strengthen new ones. In some instances, having an action plan may help you to build up evidence that contradicts your unhelpful thoughts.

The type of action plan that you make will depend on your unhelpful thoughts. Below are some ideas for action plans that may be helpful for different kinds of unhelpful thoughts.

Thoughts about not making much progress:

- Write down improvements that you have made, however small.
- Re-read relevant chapters from this book to see if there is anything else that you can do to further your improvement.
- Talk to your partner/friend/relative to see if they can help you.

Thoughts about the symptoms getting worse:

- Re-read the relevant chapters from this book.
- If you have new and severe symptoms that last for more than a few days, speak to your doctor.

Thoughts related to not achieving what you want to achieve/doing things well, etc. (Perfectionism):

- If you are focusing on a negative aspect of yourself or your situation (e.g. if you feel responsible for something that has not gone well), construct a 'responsibility pie chart'. See page 163 for an example.
- Write a list of things that you have achieved, however small.
- Set aside time to consider whether you are asking too much of yourself at present.
- Prioritise what is important to you. Can you lessen the amount that you have given yourself to do?
- Could you delegate a task/ask someone else to help?

Thoughts about not managing to do mundane tasks

- Allocate a few minutes a day or a few minutes two or three times a week to doing something that you are putting off or finding difficult.
- Plan to do something that you enjoy after your mundane task.

Thoughts related to doing something new:

- Allocate a time to buy materials for a new hobby e.g. painting.
- Allocate time each day to prepare for a course, plan how to get there, etc.
- Speak to prospective employers/tutors/course leaders/voluntary work leaders, and so on, about your concerns.
- Write down any other practical steps to help you to achieve your new goal.

Thoughts about loneliness:

- Contact old friends again.
- Explore ways of making new friends.

Thoughts about never having time for yourself:

- Prioritise 'quality' time for yourself each day, even if it's a few minutes.
- Ask others for help/delegate jobs so that you have more time for yourself.

Constructing a 'Responsibility Pie Chart'

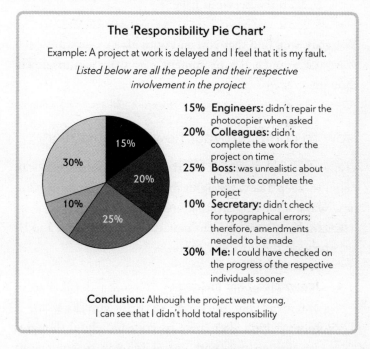

The 'Responsibility Pie Chart'

Example: A project at work is delayed and I feel that it is my fault.

Listed below are all the people and their respective involvement in the project

15% Engineers: didn't repair the photocopier when asked

20% Colleagues: didn't complete the work for the project on time

25% Boss: was unrealistic about the time to complete the project

10% Secretary: didn't check for typographical errors; therefore, amendments needed to be made

30% Me: I could have checked on the progress of the respective individuals sooner

Conclusion: Although the project went wrong, I can see that I didn't hold total responsibility

Figure 9.2 The 'Responsibility Pie Chart'

If you are focusing on a negative aspect of either yourself or a situation, it can be helpful to think about all the other people who were involved and may have affected the outcome.

- Make a list of everyone involved.
- Draw a circle and allocate them percentages according to how much responsibility you think each has for the outcome/situation, leaving yourself until last.

- See the example of a responsibility pie chart, Figure 9.2, on the previous page.

You may well find that you end up with a picture in which you take a much less prominent part than you originally thought.

How to complete your new thoughts diary

Using the steps outlined on the last few pages, you can begin to keep a new thoughts diary to help you to develop new ways of looking at situations.

Examples of two types of new thought diaries (A and B) are given on the next few pages.

- New Thoughts Diary (A). This is a detailed form where all the questions to help you look for a more helpful alternative to your unhelpful thoughts are written out, with spaces for you to enter your answers. Please see a completed diary on the next three pages, followed by a blank form for your own use.
- We find that many of our patients choose to use this form first before moving on to form B.
- New Thoughts Diary (B). This is a shorter form where you can just answer the questions on page 170 that you feel are most relevant to help you to come up with alternative thoughts. Please see instructions on how to complete this form on pages 173–4,

followed by a completed form and a blank one for your own use.

NEW THOUGHTS DIARY (A)

Situation: What was I doing at the time of my thoughts?

Talking with Jane about planning family visits.

Emotion(s): How was I feeling (angry/worried/anxious, etc.)?

Rate intensity of the feeling(s): 0–100 per cent.

Anxious: 50 per cent.

Thought(s): What thoughts went through my mind about the above situation?

Pose your thoughts as statements rather than questions, as it will be easier to come up with helpful alternatives, e.g., 'People will laugh at me', rather than 'What will people think of me?' 'I will never get better', instead of 'What if I don't get better?'

Rate your belief in the thought(s): 0–100 per cent.

I'm going to feel unwell while travelling: 50 per cent.

I'm going to feel unwell while travelling and I won't be able to do anything about it: 70 per cent.

Now that you have written down your thoughts, look through them and decide which one makes you feel worse (i.e., provokes the most emotion). Highlight that thought and base your answers to the following questions on that particular thought.

Questions

- **Am I making any thinking errors?**
  Have a look at your list of unhelpful patterns of thinking/thinking errors and write a few down.
  ° Over-generalisation.
  ° Eliminating the positive.
  ° All or nothing.

- **Have there been times in the past when I have had experiences that indicate that this thought is not true all of the time?**
  (If yes, write a few down)
  Yes. On multiple occasions, I have not felt unwell when travelling.

- **What might someone else think in this situation?**
  Another person may see a spectrum, whereas I tend to see it as black or white.

- **If my best friend or someone I loved had been in a similar situation, would I say the things that I have said to myself to him or to her? Yes or no? If no, what might I say to them?**
  No, I would be more reassuring, particularly regarding the seeming inevitability of this thought.

- **If my best friend or someone who is close knew**

that I was thinking these things, what would they say to me?

Tell me not to worry and help figure out a coping strategy or practical things we could do in the event I did feel unwell or anxious.

- **What is the actual evidence or facts that make this thought true?**

  None. I don't actually know how I'm going to feel.

- **Are there any small details or evidence that proves that this thought is wrong or not entirely accurate?**

  The feelings of ill–health could be caused by, or contributed to, by the anxiety of feeling unwell in the first place.

- **Am I blaming myself for something that wasn't entirely my fault?**

  I don't blame myself for this.

- **Am I being too self-critical and expecting too much of myself?**

  I'm possibly expecting myself to feel better than I do in this type of situation.

- **What are the advantages and disadvantages of thinking this way?**
  - Advantages: Not being overzealous when feeling well.
  - Disadvantages: Disillusionment with travel; adds anxiety that may have no basis.

- **Alternative thoughts**
  Read through your answers to the questions above and based on your answers write down a few more 'helpful' or 'balanced' thoughts.
  ° It's not a given that I'm going to feel unwell.
  ° There are things that I can do to reduce the chance of that happening.
  ° If I do feel unwell, it doesn't mean that I can't control it.

- **Outcome**
  How much do you believe your original unhelpful thought? (0–100 per cent)
  20 per cent

  What are your emotions/feelings now? How intense are they (0–100 per cent)
  20 per cent

- **Action plan**
  What can I put into place to help myself feel better in regard to the original unhelpful thought?
  Remind myself of all the positive travel experiences I've had.

  Accept the possibility I may feel unwell, but it's not a foregone conclusion and it's not black and white.

  How and when will I implement this plan?
  By talking it through with Jane, or by myself, whenever travel plans come up.

NEW THOUGHTS DIARY (A)

Situation: What was I doing at the time of my thoughts?

Emotion(s): How was I feeling? (angry/worried/anxious, etc.).

Rate intensity of the feeling(s): 0–100 per cent

Thought(s): What thoughts went through my mind about the above situation?

Pose your thoughts as statements rather than questions, as it will be easier to come up with helpful alternatives, e.g., 'People will laugh at me', rather than 'What will people think of me?' 'I will never get better', instead of 'What if I don't get better?'

Rate your belief in the thought(s): 0–100 per cent

Now that you have written down your thoughts, look through them and decide which one makes you feel the worst (i.e., provokes the most emotion). Highlight that thought and base your answers to the following questions on that particular thought.

Questions

- **Am I making any thinking errors?**
  Have a look at your list of unhelpful patterns of thinking/thinking errors and write a few down.
  - ◦
  - ◦
  - ◦

- **Have there been times in the past when I have had experiences that indicate that this thought is not true all of the time?**
  (If yes, write a few down).

- **What might someone else think in this situation?**

- **If my best friend or someone I loved had been in a similar situation, would I say the things that I have said to myself to him or to her? Yes or no? If no, what might I say to them?**

- **If my best friend or someone who is close knew that I was thinking these things, what would they say to me?**

- **What is the actual evidence or facts that make this thought true?**

- **Are there any small details or evidence that proves that this thought is wrong or not entirely accurate?**

- **Am I blaming myself for something that wasn't entirely my fault?**

- **Am I being too self-critical and expecting too much of myself?**

- **What are the advantages and disadvantages of thinking this way?**
  - Advantages:
  - Disadvantages:

- **Alternative thoughts**
  Read through your answers to the questions above and based on your answers write down a few more 'helpful' or 'balanced' thoughts.
  -
  -
  -

- **Outcome**

  How much do you believe your original unhelpful thought? (0–100 per cent)

  . . . .

  What are your emotions/feelings now? How intense are they? (0–100 per cent)

  . . . .

- **Action plan**

  What can I put into place to help myself feel better in regard to the original unhelpful thought?

     °

     °

     °

How and when will I implement this plan?

   °

NEW THOUGHTS DIARY (B)

Please see the instructions below on how to complete this diary

The first four columns of this new thoughts diary are the same as your unhelpful thoughts diary.

- Date: record the date to help you keep track of your progress.
- In the 'Situation' column, write down what you were doing or thinking about prior to having a strong feeling or change in your mood.
- In the 'Emotion' column, write down the emotion or feeling that you had at the time that you had your unhelpful thought. Rate how strong your emotion was on a 0–100 per cent scale.
- In the 'Unhelpful thoughts' column, write down the actual thought(s) that went through your mind. Rate how much you believe each thought, on a 0–100 per cent scale.
- If you have difficulty in thinking in terms of percentages, then it is fine to write down words that are meaningful to you instead.
- In the 'Evidence for and against your thoughts' column, first write down any thinking errors that you notice in your unhelpful thoughts; then write down your answers to questions that you feel are relevant on page 159.
- In the 'Alternative thoughts' column, write down

two or three alternative thoughts after reflecting on the information that you have written in the previous column. The idea is for these thoughts to be more balanced and helpful. Rate each new thought in terms of how much you believe it on a 0–100 per cent scale.

- In the 'Outcome' column, re-rate your belief in your unhelpful thoughts, and the intensity of your emotions, each on a 0–100 per cent scale. Re-rating your beliefs and emotions will indicate how helpful your alternative thoughts are. If there is little or no change in your ratings of emotions and belief in your unhelpful thought after you have come up with alternative thoughts, you may like to try to think of more alternatives or come back to it later.

- In the 'Action plan' column, write down what you can put in place to help you deal with your original unhelpful thought, improve your situation and feel better. Depending on what you come up with, it may be helpful to include time on your activity programme to carry out your action plan.

Points to bear in mind when tackling unhelpful thoughts

- Do not give up if you find the process difficult at first; like anything new, it takes practice and it can take a while for you to benefit from the process.
- It can be difficult to tackle unhelpful thoughts in

the way described above when you feel really upset, anxious, etc. However, we would suggest that you write down your unhelpful thoughts as soon as you can, so that you do not forget any details. Come back to them when you feel a little calmer, as you will be in a better position to tackle them.

- Alternative thoughts are ones that help you to change the way you *feel* about a situation or problem. They do not have to be relentlessly positive!

- It will take time and practice to build up belief in your alternative responses.

- You may find the same type of thought recurring; this is likely to happen if unhelpful thinking is well established. If this is the case, you may find Section 3 on tackling unhelpful assumptions and core beliefs to be helpful.

- After a while, you may be able to challenge your unhelpful thoughts in your head. Initially, however, writing them down will help you to be more objective.

- Remember that there is no right or wrong way of thinking. The aim of challenging your unhelpful thoughts is to help you to feel better.

New thoughts diary, example 1

Date	Situation	Emotion	Unhelpful thoughts	Evidence for and against your thoughts	Alternative thoughts	Outcome	Action plan
	What was I doing at the time of my thoughts?	How did I feel? Rate intensity (0–100 per cent).	What thoughts went through my mind just before I started to feel this way? Rate belief (0–100 per cent).	Note down thinking errors (see pages 156–8) Write answers to the questions on page 159.	Write alternative thoughts after answering questions in previous column. Rate belief in each thought (0–100 per cent).	Re-rate belief in thought and intensity (0–100 per cent).	What can I do now?
1 Jan.	Watching TV, thinking about what I had done during the day.	Frustrated (80 per cent).	I have had an awful day; I don't seem to have achieved anything (95 per cent).	Eliminating the positive. Others may say that I had managed to get up and get dressed and had done a few jobs.	Although I have not done all I planned for the day, I have done about half (90 per cent). A few weeks ago, if I had felt as	unhelpful thought (40 per cent). Emotion (40 per cent).	Praise myself for what I have achieved, rather than focusing on what I haven't done. Start afresh tomorrow.

No, I wouldn't say these things to my best friend if she were in a similar situation. I would tell her that she'd done well under the circumstances. No evidence I have done something today.	I did today. I would probably have stayed in bed all day (90 per cent).		Write a list of things that I achieve each day

New thoughts diary, example 2

Date	Situation	Emotion	Unhelpful thoughts	Evidence for and against your thoughts	Alternative thoughts	Outcome	Action plan
	What was I doing at the time of my thoughts?	How did I feel? Rate intensity (0–100 per cent).	What thoughts went through my mind just before I started to feel this way? Rate belief (0–100 per cent).	Note down thinking errors (see pages 156–8). Write answers to the questions on page 159.	Write alternative thoughts after answering questions in previous column. Rate belief in each thought (0–100 per cent).	Re-rate belief in thought and intensity (0–100 per cent).	What can I do now?
2 Jan.	Feeling ill, woke up with swollen glands.	Fed up (100 per cent).	This is never-ending (100 per cent).	Catastrophising Over-generalising Yes, I don't always feel like this. Another person may say that	I am actually much better than I was a few months ago, despite having swollen glands today (100 per cent).	Thought (65 per cent). Emotion (60 per cent).	Stick to my programme as much as possible.

178

my swollen glands are only temporary. I have no evidence that this thought is true. Maybe I am forgetting that there are times when I am feeling better.	Maybe my swollen glands are an indication that I have been doing too much lately and need to calm down a bit (80 per cent).		

New thoughts diary

Date	Situation	Emotion	Unhelpful thoughts	Evidence for and against your thoughts	Alternative thoughts	Outcome	Action plan
	What was I doing at the time of my thoughts?	How did I feel? Rate intensity (0–100 per cent).	What thoughts went through my mind just before I started to feel this way? Rate belief (0–100 per cent).	Note down thinking errors (see pages 156–8). Write answers to the questions on page 159	Write alternative thoughts after answering questions in previous column. Rate belief in each thought (0–100 per cent).	Re-rate belief in thought and intensity (0–100 per cent).	What can I do now?

Section 3:
Tackling 'unhelpful' conditional assumptions and core beliefs

Addressing your unhelpful thoughts as described in Section 2 of this chapter may be all that is necessary to help you to overcome or deal with them. However, if you find that it is more difficult to come up with more balanced alternative thoughts or you have several unhelpful thoughts based on a single theme, or thoughts come up again and again however much you challenge them, you may find this section helpful. In addition, this section may help you to better understand the reasons for recurrent problem areas in your life and help you to find ways to move forward.

It is important to say that we will all have core beliefs and assumptions that we are probably not aware of; some helpful as well as some that are not so helpful. This section is just focusing on the troublesome unhelpful ones!

When should I move on to this section?

We would suggest that you start to work through this section when you have made some progress in challenging your unhelpful thoughts.

Cautionary note

It is important for you to note, however, that this section can take weeks or months to result in any positive changes; this is because you would be working with deeper levels of cognition (assumptions and beliefs) that are generally harder to change. You may find it helpful to put half an hour or so aside to read this section through. If you feel that you would like to work through this section, be aware that you may find some of the exercises a little challenging. It may be helpful to talk to someone close to you about what you are going to be working on so that they can offer you some support, if necessary.

Levels of thoughts

We have different levels of thoughts. For our purposes here, it is useful to identify three.

Automatic thoughts

You have been addressing your automatic thoughts in the previous section of this chapter. Automatic thoughts are the most accessible level, and after some practice are fairly easy to identify. These are generally the things that we say to ourselves and that can help us to make sense of our experiences. They can be a direct reflection of our assumptions or core beliefs (for examples of these, see below) or they may be driven by them. For example, a thought such as 'I didn't do well in my exam' may be driven by a core belief 'I am not good enough'. A thought such as 'I don't have any friends' may come from a belief that 'I am not lovable'. Automatic thoughts are the easiest to change, as they are nearest the surface.

Conditional assumptions

Conditional assumptions are less obvious than our automatic thoughts and are often outside of our awareness. They operate as rules that guide our daily actions and expectations. They help us to 'get by' and to cover up perceived flaws, e.g., 'to do everything perfectly' to prevent us being criticised. They often have the force of commands such as 'I must' or 'I should', or may be posed as 'if . . . then . . .' sentences. Please see some examples of conditional assumptions below:

I should always put maximum effort into everything I do.

I *should* put others' needs first.

I *must* do everything perfectly.

If I get something wrong, *then* I would be embarrassed and fear criticism from other people.

If I'm not talkative when I go out, *then* people will think I'm boring.

If I ask for help, *then* people will think that I am weak or incompetent.

If I put others first, *then* they will like me.

The development of assumptions is influenced by our core beliefs.

Core beliefs

Core beliefs are the deepest level of thought. They are absolute statements that we hold about ourselves, other people or the world. Examples are:

I am unlovable.	*I am lovable.*
I am incompetent.	*I am OK.*
I am a failure.	*I am happy with myself.*
I am bad.	*I am good.*
Other people are better than me.	*I am as good as other people.*
Others are untrustworthy.	*Others are trustworthy.*
I am worthless.	*I am valuable.*
The world is a frightening place.	*The world is a safe place.*

Where do conditional assumptions and core beliefs come from?

The experiences that we have while growing up lead us to form conclusions (beliefs and assumptions) to help us to try to make sense of ourselves, other people and the world. If we encounter traumatic experiences – for example, bullying, abuse of any kind, or excessive criticism – we may develop negative or unhelpful core beliefs and assumptions to help us cope with our situation. It is important to note, however, that if you have had some negative experiences you will not automatically develop negative core beliefs. Some people who have encountered difficult times may develop beliefs such as 'I am a survivor', 'I am a coper', 'I am OK' when they have got through difficult times. Everyone is different. Our personality is also a factor that is likely to influence the beliefs and assumptions that we develop.

Throughout our lives, core beliefs may be activated in certain situations, resulting in our thinking, feeling and behaving in ways that may further exacerbate unhelpful thoughts and feelings. (Please see Figure 9.3 on the next page for a diagram showing how this can work.)

Unhelpful core beliefs that we acquire as young children are unlikely to be true, but we take them as such until we are able to be more flexible in our thinking. For example, if a young child is scratched or bitten by a dog, they may think that all dogs are dangerous and be frightened of them. It is unlikely that they will change their attitude about them until they are older; then, when they see friends playing with dogs, they may learn that some dogs are friendly, and some dogs are not.

When we get older, not only do we generally learn to be more flexible in our rules and beliefs, we also learn to change our behaviour according to the situation. For example, we usually learn that it is safe to approach a dog that is wagging its tail, but not to approach one that is growling.

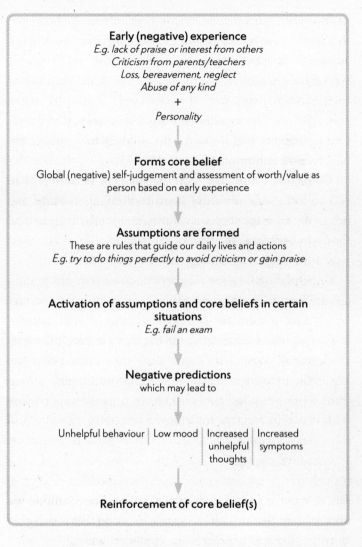

Figure 9.3 The formation of (negative) core beliefs and possible consequences

Some of the 'negative' beliefs we develop in childhood may stay with us into adulthood. There may be a number of reasons, which include:

- Experiencing trauma of any kind.
- Repeatedly facing situations that reinforce the beliefs. For example, a child who is constantly being criticised at home and/or at school might conclude that he/she is bad and develop the core belief of being 'bad', 'a failure'/'not good enough'. This belief may then be reinforced later in life: for example, getting lower marks than expected in exams, an unsuccessful job application, being criticised at work or by friends.
- Ongoing 'negative' experiences, such as observing a 'successful' sibling or friends at school who receive much praise, can lead to the development of 'unhelpful' core beliefs about others; for example, 'others are more competent/better than me'. This belief can then reinforce negative beliefs about oneself, such as 'I'm not good enough'. Other negative experiences, such as trauma, bullying or rejection, can also lead to unhelpful beliefs about others such as 'others are untrustworthy'.

Because our core beliefs help us to make sense of the world at a young age, it rarely occurs to us to assess whether they are the most useful ways of understanding our adult experiences. Instead, we tend to go on acting, thinking and feeling as if these beliefs were true. Also, although many core beliefs stem from childhood, we can acquire new negative core beliefs at any age, through powerful negative experiences such as witnessing or experiencing trauma; living in chaotic, unpredictable circumstances; or experiencing persistent unhappiness for whatever reason.

What are the effects of holding negative core beliefs?

Negative or unhelpful core beliefs lead to negative consequences in terms of how we think, feel and behave. When we have asked patients directly about consequences of beliefs such as 'I'm not good enough', they have reported consequences such as 'feeling restricted', 'stressed', 'watching over my shoulder for the next mistake', 'avoiding trying new things', 'feel bad about myself', 'don't like myself'. These negative consequences arise because of harsh rules and strategies that people put into place to cope with their belief.

Let us share with you Sarah's example.

Background information

Sarah had always felt that her mum had had high expectations of her and that her father tended to be critical of her, particularly for speaking quietly. Sarah moved schools a few times and felt a pressure to do well from her teachers, herself and her parents. She felt too shy to ask for help or be able to make friends.

Unhelpful core belief

I am not good enough.

Assumptions

Rules that guide your behaviour:

'If I don't do well, I'll let other people down.'

'If I'm late, people might get annoyed.'

'If people shout/get cross with me, it upsets me and makes me feel bad.'

'If people like my clothes, they will like me.'

Compensatory strategies

Behaviours that help you cope with your belief:

Avoiding doing new things; working really hard.

Planning to get to places early.

Trying to avoid being shouted at, e.g., by speaking louder.

Trying to please people, e.g. by buying great gifts.

Trying to impress/compensate by wearing particular clothes.

Typical situations in which my rules and behaviours may become activated

When I have been invited to a social event.

Prior to an exam or meeting deadlines.

Prior to leaving home to meet people.

Unhelpful automatic thoughts and emotions

'If I don't do well, I'll let other people down' (stress).

'If people like my clothes, they will like me' (anxious).

'If I'm late, people may get annoyed' (anxious).

Behaviour in response to thoughts

Staying in my room/avoidance of event.

Studying until I'm exhausted.

Preparing for hours to get ready.

Planning journeys well in advance and checking the journey the night before and on the day.

A consequence of Sarah's harsh rules and compensatory strategies was that she often felt stressed because of putting so much pressure on herself. This exacerbated her fatigue and made it difficult to complete her work for her degree as well as to socialise.

What is the point in trying to challenge assumptions and core beliefs?

Challenging your negative core beliefs and assumptions is likely to lead to a number of benefits that may include:

- fewer unhelpful thoughts;
- a gradual decline in the amount you believe your negative core belief;

- rules becoming less harsh, leading to less pressure on yourself to do achieve high standards, do things perfectly etc.;
- reduced stress/feeling upset, etc.;
- putting less pressure on yourself, which may help to reduce fatigue and other symptoms.

As the strength of your core belief lessens, you will be on a path to be able to identify a more helpful core belief. You may also set less harsh rules for yourself, which will help you to adopt new ways of behaving (strategies) that are more consistent with your new, 'helpful' core beliefs. For example, you may be willing to accept small mistakes, be pleased about things that you achieve, and be more inclined to take risks and to try new things. In addition, you may find it easier to prioritise yourself and take time to relax and do enjoyable things.

You can see Sarah's new belief, rules and strategies that she came up with after a few months of her challenging her unhelpful core belief on pages 213–14.

How do I identify assumptions and core beliefs about myself?

There are a couple of ways to identify core beliefs; have a read through them both to see which you think you may find most helpful.

1. Identify themes from your unhelpful thoughts

Look back at some of the 'unhelpful thoughts' you wrote

down in the thought diaries that you completed in the last section. Do you notice any common themes? If so, they may provide you with some clues. For example, if you notice that a lot of your unhelpful thoughts are related to being critical of yourself, your theme may be to do with being not good enough/a failure/incompetent, etc. If a number of thoughts are related to feeling left out/rejected by others, a theme may be about not being liked or not being lovable.

If you are unable to find a particular theme from looking at your unhelpful thoughts, then you may find the second technique more helpful. This is what we call the 'downward arrow' technique.

2. The downward arrow technique

- First, find an unhelpful thought about yourself in your unhelpful thoughts diary or new thoughts diary, one that was associated with an intense emotion.
- Write down the situation where you had the unhelpful thought, and the thought itself. Then ask yourself: '*What does this say or mean about me?*'
- Keep asking this question of each answer you come up with until you arrive at a core belief about yourself.
- You may only need to ask the above question once or twice to arrive at a core belief; on the other hand, you may need to ask it three or four times.

Here is an example of how a core belief is identified using the downward arrow technique.

Example of an unhelpful core belief about me

Situation	**You are called in to see your boss at work.**
Thought	*He doesn't think my work is good enough; I'm bound to get the sack.*

Question	What does this say or mean about me?
Answer	*I'm no good at my job.*

Question	What does this say or mean about me?
Answer	*I'm no good at anything.*

Question	What does this say or mean about me?
Answer	*I am incompetent – core belief.*

A blank copy of an 'Identifying core beliefs' worksheet setting out this process is provided on page 196 for you to photocopy and fill in.

Identifying and challenging core beliefs about yourself may be enough to help you feel better about things in addition to understanding a recurrent problem in your life. However, identifying and challenging unhelpful core beliefs about others, too, may help you to get things into better perspective. For example, having a core belief that 'everyone is more competent than me' could compound a core belief about being 'incompetent'. If you are able to challenge this belief and identify a new belief such as 'others are not competent all the time', this may help you to feel less 'incompetent'.

How do I identify core beliefs about other people?

You can identify core beliefs connected with other people using the same guidelines given for identifying core beliefs about yourself. Instead of using an unhelpful thought about yourself, find one that is about other people. Again, a blank worksheet is provided on page 198.

EXAMPLE OF AN UNHELPFUL CORE BELIEF ABOUT OTHER PEOPLE

Situation:	**You are at a get–together with old school friends. They are all talking about what they have been doing.**
Thought	*They all lead far more interesting lives than me.*
Question	What does this say or mean about other people?
Answer	*They are more interesting than me.*
Question	What does this say or mean about other people?
Answer	*They are better than me.*
Question	What does this say or mean about me?
Answer	*Other people are better than me – core belief.*

WORKSHEET: IDENTIFYING CORE BELIEFS ABOUT ME

Situation: _____

_____

_____

Unhelpful thought: _____

_____

Question: *What does this say or mean about me?*

Answer: _____

_____

Question: *What does this say or mean about me?*

Answer: _____

_____

Question: *What does this say or mean about me?*

Answer: _____

_____

Question: *What does this say or mean about me?*

Core belief: _____

_____

_____

WORKSHEET: IDENTIFYING CORE BELIEFS ABOUT OTHER PEOPLE

Situation: _____

_____

_____

Unhelpful thought: _____

_____

Question: *What does this say or mean about others?*

Answer: _____

_____

Question: *What does this say or mean about others?*

Answer: _____

_____

Question: *What does this say or mean about others?*

Answer: _____

_____

Question: *What does this say or mean about others?*

Core belief: _____

_____

_____

Now that you have identified a core belief(s), you may find it helpful to try to understand where they have come from and the effects they have on you. The chart on the next page gives an example of how a person's core belief may be formed and maintained. A blank version of the chart is given on pages 201–2 so you can fill in an example of your own, if you wish. You can also refer to Sarah's example of an unhelpful core belief on pages 181–91.

Thinking about experiences you had while growing up can help you to understand the origins and make sense of your core beliefs. However, focusing on this background information can sometimes be upsetting or distressing; particularly if you have encountered traumatic or difficult experiences in your life. If this is the case, we would recommend that you do not spend too long on this section. Also, you may find it helpful to talk about what you are doing with someone close to you to gain some support.

For the purposes of tackling your core beliefs and assumptions, complete the boxes labelled 'core belief', 'assumptions' and 'strategies'. For you to develop a better understanding of how your beliefs and assumptions affect you, it will be helpful for you to complete the bottom four boxes.

Example of how core beliefs may be formed and maintained

Background information
What experiences contributed to the development and maintenance of the core belief?

Criticism from parents.

Comparison with my older sister who was cleverer than me.

Failing my 11+.

Being bullied at primary and secondary school.

Unhelpful core belief
What is my most unhelpful core belief?

I am a failure.

Assumptions
*Rules that guide my behaviour
(usually expressed as 'if . . . then' statements)*

If I don't do well at something then there's no point in doing it.

I should always do my best whatever the cost.

If I ask for help, it is a sign of weakness.

If my house is untidy then people will think I'm lazy.

Strategies that maintain my core belief

Avoidance of trying new things.

Have very high standards; spending a lot of time checking work, etc.

Work very hard; over-prepare.

Avoid asking for help.

Spending a lot of time cleaning the house, preparing for guests.

Typical situations in which my rules and beliefs may be activated

a. If I am asked to do something new at work/or a friend suggests trying a new activity.

b. Preparing for friends to come round.

c. Reviewing a piece of my own work.

d. Meeting new people.

Unhelpful automatic thoughts (and emotions)
that may occur in the above situations and reinforce core belief

a. I'm sure I won't be good at this (worried).

b. They will think that my house is really messy (anxious).

c. I should be able to understand this. My supervisor will think I'm really stupid if I say I'm stuck (upset)!

d. I've nothing interesting to say (worried).

Behaviour in response to thoughts

a. Try to avoid it/make excuses/delay activity.

b. Spend excessive time cleaning/tidying.

c. Check work again, put off asking for help unless absolutely necessary.

d. Keep quiet.

How core beliefs may be formed and maintained

Background information
*What experiences contributed to the development and
maintenance of the core belief?*

_____

_____

_____

Unhelpful core belief
What is my most unhelpful core belief?

_____

_____

_____

Assumptions
*Rules that guide my behaviour
(usually expressed as 'if . . . then' statements)*

_____

_____

_____

Strategies that maintain my core belief

_____

_____

_____

Typical situations in which my rules and beliefs may be activated

_____

_____

_____

Unhelpful automatic thoughts (and emotions)
*that may occur in the above situations and
reinforce core belief*

_____

_____

_____

Behaviour in response to thoughts

_____

_____

_____

Contesting core beliefs

As we have already mentioned, unhelpful core beliefs can take a lot longer to change than unhelpful thoughts, because we require a lot more convincing that these deeper-held beliefs are not true.

To give yourself an idea of how much you believe your core belief(s), have a look at the example below. Then, in the space(s) provided, write your own core belief(s) and put an X on the line to represent how strong your belief is.

CORE BELIEF

I am unlovable

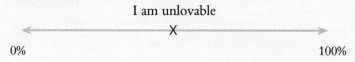

0%   100%

CORE BELIEF

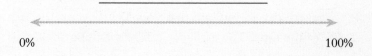

0%   100%

CORE BELIEF

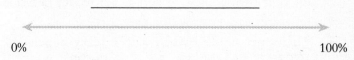

0%   100%

Generally speaking, the stronger the belief, the more work you will have to do to challenge it. However, with persistence you can get there. Take Sarah as an example: she really could not imagine feeling differently about herself when she began her core belief work, but after a couple of months, she began to feel a lot better.

Remember, you have already learned how to challenge your unhelpful thoughts, so you will have acquired techniques that will help you to question the accuracy of your core beliefs.

There are two main ways of contesting core beliefs:

1. Finding evidence to challenge your belief (see below).
2. Conducting your own behavioural experiments to test the accuracy of your existing thoughts, assumptions and core beliefs (please see pages 207–8).

Finding evidence to challenge a core belief

- Try to find at least one or two pieces of evidence every day to indicate that your belief is not true all of the time. The evidence can be anything at all; the examples in the 'contesting core belief record' boxes on page 206 may give you some ideas.
- Each day, write down your piece(s) of evidence on your own contesting core belief record (a blank record sheet is provided on page 209).
- There may be days when it feels really difficult to come up with any evidence at all. This may be because you don't feel that you have done much, something has gone wrong or you are just feeling

really unwell. On these occasions, it may be helpful for you to think about what a friend or someone close to you may say about your day, or what you may say to a friend.

- When you are able to find a piece of evidence most days that refutes your belief, try to find two or three pieces of evidence each day.
- When you have a list of about twenty to thirty items, look at them and draw your own conclusions about whether your original core belief accurately describes your whole experience.
- You may also find it helpful to look back at the X on your line where you rated your strength of belief and put another X on the line with today's date to see how much things have changed. If you feel that your rating has not changed, or only changed a little, do not give up. Keep going with finding evidence to challenge your belief every day and then have a look at your rating in a few weeks' time.
- When you no longer feel that your unhelpful core belief accurately describes your situation or how you feel (this might be after a few weeks or months), then turn to pages 212–14 to find out how to identify a new and more helpful core belief.

Please see below examples of evidence that you could write to challenge a core belief of 'I am not good enough'.

CONTESTING CORE BELIEF RECORD, EXAMPLE 1

Unhelpful core belief: I am not good enough.

Evidence or experiences that indicate that my core belief is not always true:

1. I got out of bed even though I didn't feel like it.
2. I enjoyed talking to my neighbour this morning.
3. I walked up a flight of stairs today; the first time in months.
4. I was complimented on a new dress that I was wearing.
5. I made meringues – a bit chewy but people seemed to enjoy them.

CONTESTING CORE BELIEF RECORD, EXAMPLE 2

Unhelpful core belief: I am not lovable.

Evidence or experiences that indicate that my core belief is not always true:

1. Charlie gave me a big hug.
2. I received a text from an old friend.
3. My neighbour called in to see how I was feeling today.
4. An assistant in the local shop said it was nice to see me again.
5. My aunt phoned to see if she could call in for a coffee as she was passing by.

2. Behavioural experiments

You can conduct your own behavioural experiments in everyday situations to test the validity of your thoughts, assumptions and beliefs.

There are different types of experiments and you may choose the one(s) that you feel will be most helpful.

- *Surveys* – can be used to gather information. So, for example, if you are challenging a belief of 'not being good enough' and one of your strategies is to spend a lot of time on a particular activity such as cleaning, or writing emails or essays, to make them 'perfect', you could ask some friends how long they spend on these activities. You can then draw your own conclusions from the results of your survey and possibly plan another experiment. So, for example, if they spend a lot less time on a particular activity than you do, you could plan an *experiential exercise* to test out your thoughts of spending less time on an activity.

- *Experiential exercises* – can be used to test specific thoughts, assumptions and beliefs, e.g. if your **core belief** is that you are 'unlikeable', you might contact friends and suggest going out/invite them for a coffee. You could make a prediction of what you think may happen and then draw your own conclusions from the results of your experiment. If you have a core belief that 'I am never good enough', which leads you to put 100 per cent effort into everything that you do, try to put slightly less effort in and see what happens. For example, if you spend on average one hour cleaning the kitchen, try spending three-quarters of an hour; again, you could predict what you think will happen. Then see what actually does happen. Has anyone noticed? Is the kitchen really that much different? Did you have more time for relaxation?

- You can also use your assumptions/rules to design experiments; so, for example, if your rule is along the lines of 'If I ask for help then people will think I'm incompetent', you could design an experiment, such as to ask for help with the cooking/cleaning/piece of work. You could make a prediction of what you think will happen and then draw your own conclusions after you've carried out your experiment.

- You could experiment with something that you perform frequently – for example, initiating a conversation every day to see how someone responds (to challenge a belief that you are unlikeable) – or with something that you do less often – for example, doing less preparation for a seminar (to challenge a belief that you are not good enough).

- As well as being a useful way to challenge unhelpful thoughts, beliefs and assumptions, behavioural experiments may also be used to help you strengthen more helpful thoughts, assumptions and core beliefs.

Please see an example of one of Sarah's behavioural experiments on page 210.

You can use the behavioural experiment record on page 211 for your own use.

CONTESTING CORE BELIEF RECORD

Unhelpful core belief: _____

Evidence or experiences that indicate that my core belief is not always true:

1. _____
2. _____
3. _____
4. _____
5. _____
6. _____
7. _____
8. _____
9. _____
10. _____
11. _____
12. _____
13. _____
14. _____
15. _____
16. _____
17. _____
18. _____
19. _____
20. _____

Conclusion:_____

_____

Sarah's example: Behavioural experiment record

Date	Thought/belief to be tested Write down the thought or belief that you want to test out.	Experiment Write down details of the actual experiment.	Prediction What do you think will happen?	Outcome of experiment What actually happened?	What have I learned from this experiment?
7th April	People will think my painting is rubbish.	Paint once a week and show my mum, no matter how bad the painting is.	She will be disappointed.	She was impressed with my drawing and said she was looking forward to seeing my next one.	Be more free and less precise and focused on it being perfect. It's just a sketch!
12th April:				Mum gave me help where I was stuck. Gave me a compliment – told me it was going well.	Practise to get better. Don't be afraid to show unfinished work. Ask for help.

210

Behavioural experiment record

Date	Thought/belief to be tested Write down the thought or belief that you want to test out.	Experiment Write down details of the actual experiment.	Prediction What do you think will happen?	Outcome of experiment What actually happened?	What have I learned from this experiment?

Identifying a new belief

It is time to move on to identifying a new belief when you feel that your 'unhelpful' core belief(s) no longer truly reflects how you feel about yourself and/or others). As we have mentioned, it may take you a few weeks or months to reach this stage. It can be a little challenging to come up with a new core belief statement, particularly when you have been stuck with an unhelpful old core belief for some time.

A new core belief may be the *opposite* of the old unhelpful core belief. For example:

Old belief: *I am unlikeable.*

New belief: I am likeable.

Old belief: *I am incompetent.*

New belief: *I am competent.*

This does not mean that you have to be likeable/competent to everyone, or all of the time.

On the other hand, you may come up with a generally more compassionate statement as an alternative to an unhelpful belief, e.g.

Old belief: *I am not good enough/a failure/incompetent.*

New belief: *I am happy with myself/I am content in myself/I am OK.*

Alternatively, a new core belief may change an absolute belief to a qualified belief. For example:

Old belief: *Everyone is better than me.*

New belief: *Not everyone is better than me; I am better than some people at certain things.*

Constructing alternative assumptions/rules and strategies

- Once you have identified your new belief(s), it is time to identify some alternative assumptions/rules and strategies to support your new belief. These rules should be more helpful, flexible and realistic.
- You can then consider strategies that will support your alternative rules.

Please see Sarah's example below.

New core belief

I am happy with myself.

Rules/assumptions to support belief

If I fail, it is not the end of the world.

If someone does not like me, it does not mean I am a bad person.

If I try something new/an old talent, I do not have to be instantly good at it.

It's OK to feel anxious at times.

I am proud of myself.

Strategies to support new belief

Accepting that I have done as much as I can.

Asking people for help/to move if necessary (on a bus), eating in public.

Doing something I enjoy even if I am not very good at it.

Acknowledging my anxiety.

Speak to more people.

You can see how much more flexible and realistic Sarah's rules and strategies are. As indicated earlier, she felt that the advantages of holding her new belief were as follows:

- I feel happier.
- Calmer.
- Less stressed and anxious.
- More likely to do more things and things I want to do.
- More confident.

A blank chart for you to use can be found on the next page.

NEW CORE BELIEF

_____

_____

_____

_____

Rules/assumptions to support belief _____

_____

_____

_____

_____

_____

Strategies to support new belief _____

_____

_____

_____

_____

_____

Advantages of holding this belief _____

_____

_____

_____

_____

_____

_____

How do I strengthen my new core belief?

1. Find evidence to support your alternative belief.
2. Carry out behavioural experiments to evaluate your new assumptions.

1. Find evidence to support your new belief

Just as you recorded evidence to indicate that your old 'unhelpful' core belief was not true all of the time, it is important that you find evidence to support and strengthen your belief in your new core belief. You can do this using the 'New core belief record' on page 217.

- First, write out your new core belief in the space provided.
- Then, over the coming weeks, try to record small events and experiences that occur each day that support your new belief. The things that you write down will be very similar to things that you wrote down on your 'contesting core beliefs record'.
- You may also like to record events and positive experiences from your past that support your new belief.

Here are a few examples from Sarah's new core belief record:

New core belief

I am happy with myself

Evidence or experience that support the new belief

I did some work on my essay even though I didn't feel like it.

I travelled via a route that I've never travelled before.

I can exercise more than I used to (a few months ago).

I cooked a really nice meal for my boyfriend.

I took time to rest and see friends.

2. Behavioural experiments

Conducting behavioural experiments can help you to test your new assumptions which in turn can help to strengthen your new beliefs and build confidence in your strategies to support your new belief. You can use the form on page 211 to plan your experiments.

Points to bear in mind about tackling core beliefs

- Reducing your belief in 'unhelpful' core beliefs often takes a long time because they may have developed and been reinforced over a long period. Don't be surprised if it takes a lot of time and patience.
- Go at your own pace; do not rush this section.
- Developing and strengthening your new core beliefs can also take time, as you may initially have difficulty in finding experiences that are consistent with them.

NEW CORE BELIEF RECORD

New core belief: _____

Evidence or experiences that support my new core belief:

1. _____
2. _____
3. _____
4. _____
5. _____
6. _____
7. _____
8. _____
9. _____
10. _____
11. _____
12. _____
13. _____
14. _____
15. _____
16. _____
17. _____
18. _____
19. _____
20. _____

- There will be times in your life when you feel greater levels of distress; at these times, you can expect to have more unhelpful thoughts, and your unhelpful core belief(s) may return. At these times, review all of your work from this chapter and repeat any of the worksheets necessary to help you to challenge your unhelpful thinking patterns and strengthen your new beliefs.

If this all feels like hard work, don't despair: it will be worth it in the long run!

10

Overcoming worry, stress and anxiety related to your chronic fatigue

This chapter aims to help you to overcome worries, stress or anxiety that you may experience from time to time in your journey to get better.

We have already discussed how having fatigue associated with CFS or another long-standing illness can at times be very stressful. Not only are you trying to cope with your illness, but you may also be dealing with other challenges, such as financial difficulties or family concerns. Trying to overcome your fatigue and other symptoms as described in this book can be challenging and at times stressful. Not only are you changing your routine; you are also filling in diaries, and maybe, at times, having a temporary increase in your symptoms.

In addition, you may be trying to resume some of your previous activities and be considering some new enterprises, such as a part-time job, a course or contacting old friends again.

Although you may be pleased to be in this position, you may naturally feel a little worried or daunted by the prospect of these changes.

Do you remember Alison, who we discussed earlier in the book? She made excellent progress in the first couple of months. She almost reached her walking target of twenty minutes twice daily, had taken over the cooking at home again as well as a few more of the household chores, and had gradually cut down some of her resting time. Her sleep had improved as a result of doing more in the day and developing a good pre-sleep routine.

However, about halfway through her sessions, she felt she had reached a plateau. When this was explored further, it transpired that the targets she had been working on thus far had felt 'comfortable', but the next step involved her thinking about doing a course, which caused her a variety of worries. Her worries were discussed at some length and she was reassured that it was completely normal to feel anxious about doing something that she had not done for a long time. It turned out that Alison had always felt a little anxious with new people and remembered being shy as a child and having some difficulties with mixing with other children. A variety of ways to help her to overcome this 'block' were discussed. First, the effects of anxiety were discussed, in terms of thoughts, behaviour and physical feelings (symptoms). It seemed that attending a college course was a more difficult target to achieve than she had originally thought. Therefore, steps were agreed to help her work towards going to college later that year. Exposure therapy was discussed as a helpful way to reduce anxiety. A list of 'easy' to 'difficult' things that she would need to be able to do in order to go to college were agreed. She was encouraged to include a few of these things in her activity programme over the next few weeks. Examples included phoning two friends every week and organising quotes for two rooms to be decorated. When she achieved these things, she was encouraged to continue working through her list. She tackled her unhelpful 'anxious' thoughts by generating helpful alternatives. Over the next few weeks she began to feel more confident in her ability to get on with people.

Questions people frequently ask themselves when trying to resume some of their previous activities or considering new enterprises include:

- 'Will I be able to do the work?'
- 'What if I can't cook a meal any more?'
- 'How will I cope with meeting new people at college for the first time when I haven't met anyone new for so long?'
- 'How will I cope on the train? I haven't travelled alone for ages.'
- 'How will I get on with my old friends? I haven't seen them for such a long time.'

Asking oneself these questions is perfectly normal, because when we haven't done things for a while or don't practise something regularly, we tend to lose confidence in our own ability, and often when we try new things we are naturally apprehensive.

These worries may sometimes trigger feelings of anxiety. We have already discussed some of the effects of anxiety in the section of Chapter 1 on 'Autonomic arousal in chronic fatigue syndrome'. Figures 10.1 and 10.2 provide further illustrations of how anxiety can affect us.

Common physical signs of extreme worry and anxiety

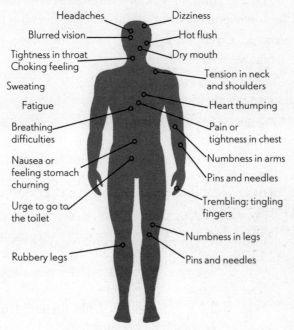

Headaches

Blurred vision

Tightness in throat
Choking feeling

Sweating

Fatigue

Breathing
difficulties

Nausea or
feeling stomach
churning

Urge to go to
the toilet

Rubbery legs

Dizziness

Hot flush

Dry mouth

Tension in neck
and shoulders

Heart thumping

Pain or
tightness in chest

Numbness in arms

Pins and needles

Trembling: tingling
fingers

Numbness in legs

Pins and needles

Some of these feelings may come on when you are extremely worried or anxious. Some may last a short time (e.g. heart thumping or breathlessness); others may persist when you no longer feel anxious (e.g. headaches, tension in neck and shoulders).

Figure 10.1 Common physical signs of
extreme worry and anxiety

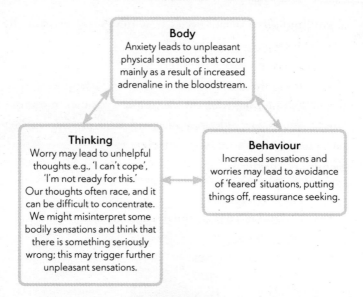

Figure 10.2 How anxiety affects our body, thoughts and behaviour

Common worries associated with chronic fatigue

Listed below are worries that people who have chronic fatigue commonly report:

Resuming previous activities/responsibilities

- Going back to work.
- Walking outside the house.
- Doing the shopping.
- Managing the home.

- Driving.
- Making contact with old friends.
- Cooking.
- Doing the shopping.
- Visiting friends.
- Travelling longer distances.

Starting a new activity

- A new job.
- A course at college/university.
- Going to the gym.
- Making new friends.

Dealing with symptoms/body sensations

- How to interpret/understand the meaning of symptoms.
- What to do about them.
- How to get the activity level 'right'.
- How to deal with a 'bad' day.

Benefits/disability allowances

- Loss of benefits leading to financial concerns.
- Dealing with the appeals process.

Difficulty in making big or small decisions

- Whether to return to the same job/go part time or apply for a new one.

- Whether going away for a weekend would be counterproductive.
- How to manage going to an event such as a wedding/theatre trip, etc.

Not knowing what to tell prospective employers

- Whether to tell prospective employers about chronic fatigue problems or not.
- Whether to ask for help/support from employers.
- Whether to discuss changing/reducing hours at work.

Feeling responsible or blaming oneself for the illness and the effect that it has on others

- If life has changed considerably e.g. a partner does all the domestic chores as well as working.
- If you are not able to do as much as previously with your partner.
- If there are reduced earnings within the family, leading to financial difficulties.
- If children are not having as much attention as they used to do.
- If colleagues have had to take on some of your work.

How to deal with your worries

In the previous chapter, we discussed challenging unhelpful thoughts and beliefs that may have helped you to deal with some of your worries. However, in this section we are going to suggest two different ways, both tried and tested, of helping you to address your worries.

A. Problem solving
B. Exposure to situations that make you anxious

We suggest that before embarking on either of them you spend a while reading through the chapter to help you to decide whether either or both strategies would be helpful.

Step 1: write any situations or activities that worry you in the space provided below

1. _____

2. _____

3. _____

4. _____

5. _____

6. _____

7. _____

Step 2: look at your list and decide what you would like to tackle first
It may be helpful if you start by tackling the things that cause you the least worry, and then move on to the more difficult situations as you gain confidence.

Step 3: decide whether a or b (below) is the best way of helping you to tackle each of your difficulties

(You may decide to use different strategies for different worries.)

A: Problem solving: this is a process that can help you to deal with practical worries.

B: Exposure to situations that make you anxious: this is a process that can help you to gradually face situations that make you feel anxious.

Step 4: include time to tackle your difficulties when you write your next activity programme.

A: Problem solving

Define the problem

What is your problem? Try to define it as clearly and objectively as possible and write it down so you can easily follow the steps outlined below to solve it. Working through a problem as described below can take some time, but is usually helpful. If you feel stuck identifying a precise problem statement, you may find it helpful to have a chat with a friend or partner about it. Other people can be more objective and may be able to help you identify the problem more clearly.

Propose alternative solutions

Think of at least three alternative ways of solving the problem. This is important, as the first solution you think of may not be the best one.

If you have difficulty thinking of any alternative solutions:

- Try to see the problem from someone else's point of view by asking the question, 'If _ _ were in my shoes, what would he or she do?'
- Use the point of view of someone who you feel has dealt well with a similar problem, or someone you feel is good at solving problems.
- Try to think about how you solved a similar problem in the past.
- Think about how you may advise a friend.

Evaluate your alternative solutions

Once you have thought of as many alternative solutions as possible, the next step is to evaluate the possible outcome(s) of each one. Do this by writing down what you think the *positive* and *negative* consequence(s) of each of your alternative solutions might be.

Make a decision

Now that you have considered the possible outcome of each solution, it's time to make a decision about which solution to the problem seems to be the best. You may find that there is more than one solution that will help you solve your problem.

Make a plan and implement the solution(s)

This stage will vary according to the type of problem you are trying to solve. It may be that no planning is needed, as it just involves saying something to someone; on the other hand, you may need to make a detailed plan of action in several stages.

Evaluate your plan

Once you have tackled your problem, ask yourself the following questions:

- Did I follow my plan in tackling the problem?
- Did the outcome that I expected to occur happen?
- Am I satisfied with the outcome?
- Would I use the same strategy/strategies again? If not, what would I do differently?

Once you have used the problem-solving technique a few times, you may be able to solve future problems in your head without the need to write anything down.

Please see the two examples of problem solving below, followed by a blank problem-solving sheet for you to photocopy and use.

PROBLEM SOLVING IN ACTION: EXAMPLE (1)

Problem definition

Difficulty coping with inconsiderate lodger.

Alternative solutions (Think of at least three)	*Evaluation of alternative solutions* (What are possible outcomes of each alternative solution?)
1. Put up with it.	1. I need the money from rent. Inactivity is unlikely to help.
2. Ask him to leave and find a new home.	2. Next lodger may be no better. May not find one for a while, which would lead to money problems.
3. Discuss problems with him.	3. This will kill or cure the problem.

Decision on best solution

3. Discuss problems with him.

Make a detailed plan

When he returns home from work, say that I would like to speak to him at his convenience.

Discuss the points that I find difficult about him.

Agree that we can review the situation again in six weeks.

Evaluation of plan

Worked well. Agreed to speak in six weeks' time.

PROBLEM SOLVING IN ACTION: EXAMPLE (2)

Problem definition

Worried about how I will cope at college, whether I will be able to keep up with the work.

Alternative solutions (Think of at least three)	*Evaluation of alternative solutions* (What are possible outcomes of each alternative solution?)
1. Speak to tutor about my problems.	1. May help my tutor to understand my difficulties and be sympathetic if I am unable to meet deadlines. But it may make me feel different from others. Do I want that?
2. Put off the course for a few months.	2. Although I may feel a little better then, I may not be that much better, and I would still have to face the problem at some time.
3. Ensure a well-balanced programme with planned study time and a mixture of activities and relaxation.	3. This will ensure that I work steadily at my coursework as well as have time for other activities and relaxation. Be prepared to be more tired initially.

Decision on best solution

3: Ensure a well-balanced programme with planned study time and a mixture of activities and relaxation.

Make a detailed plan

Find out at college how much coursework I will be expected to do each week/term.

Review my current activity programme and include regular time for studying. Try to study for short times frequently rather than for long periods occasionally.

Ensure that my programme includes a mixture of activities with relaxation time.

Evaluation of plan

It will not be immediately clear whether my solution was the best one, as it is likely that I will be more tired initially when I start my course (as with any new activity). Review the situation after a couple of weeks and amend my activity programme, if necessary.

If, after a month, I feel that I am struggling, then it may be helpful to discuss my difficulties with my tutor.

PROBLEM SOLVING IN ACTION	
Problem definition	
Alternative solutions (Think of at least three)	*Evaluation of alternative solutions* (What are possible outcomes of each alternative solution?)
1.	1.
2.	2.
3.	3.
4.	4.
Decision on best solution	
Make a detailed plan	
Evaluation of plan	

B: Exposure to situations that cause anxiety

If you have had CFS or another health problem causing fatigue for a long time, it is likely that you will have stopped some activities or got out of practice at doing certain things. These may be small things, such as taking responsibility for paying the household expenses, or making phone calls; or they may be bigger things, such as driving a car, giving a presentation at work or having people round for a meal. If you stop things or don't practise them regularly, it's easy to lose confidence in yourself – and this can happen quite quickly.

We have all been in situations where we have felt anxious initially: for example, meeting new people, our first day at school, college or work, getting married, attending interviews, etc. However, after a few minutes of being in an 'anxiety-provoking' situation such as the examples above, we usually start to feel better and are able to concentrate on the matter at hand; this is because anxiety naturally reduces over time. 'Exposure therapy' makes use of this fact and can be a very effective way of overcoming anxiety. It involves repeatedly confronting situations that make you feel anxious and staying in the situation until the anxiety subsides.

The following guidelines aim to help you overcome anxiety in specific situations.

Write a list of all the situations that cause you anxiety

- Have a look at the list of situations that you wrote down on pages 227–8.
- Write them in order from the *least* difficult to the *most* difficult, and start with the one that causes you the *least* anxiety.

Plan specific exposure tasks to do at regular times and as frequently as possible

- Write down the exposure tasks in your activity programme. The tasks that you choose will obviously depend on the situation that makes you feel anxious.
- For example, if you have lost confidence in your ability to socialise and have lost contact with most of your friends, you may decide to start facing this challenge by phoning a friend three times a week. Once you feel that you are managing this exposure task with little anxiety, then you can move on to the next step on your list, which may be to have a friend round or meet with a friend for an hour or so per week.
- On the other hand, you may have stopped doing a lot of activities at home that have now been taken over by your partner. You may decide, when you are feeling well enough, to gradually take some of these activities over, e.g., by sharing the cooking, then cooking for your family, and then inviting friends over and cooking a meal for them. You may gradually

introduce doing the shopping, making phone calls, paying bills, etc.

Expect to feel anxious

When confronting situations that you have not encountered for some time, it is likely that you will feel anxious for a while; as we mentioned earlier, this is perfectly normal. Remember that these feelings are nothing more than an exaggeration of quite normal bodily reactions to stress.

How to manage your anxiety in an anxiety-provoking situation

It's all very well us asking you to stay in an 'anxiety-provoking' situation until you feel better, but we thought that it may help if we gave you some tips on how to do this!

- Stay in the situation until your anxiety subsides.
- Although feeling anxious is uncomfortable, it is not harmful. Wait and give the anxiety time to pass without fighting it or running away from it.
- Speak calmly to yourself. Remind yourself that you can do this.
- Tell yourself that any bodily sensations you experience are nothing more than a normal reaction to stress.
- If you notice changes with your breathing when anxious, then the breathing exercises outlined on the next page may be helpful.

Diaphragmatic breathing exercises

When people are scared or very anxious, they often breathe more shallowly and rapidly and use their upper lungs. Breathing in this way is referred to as 'hyperventilation' and can lead to uncomfortable feelings such as dizziness, shortness of breath, nausea and tingling or numbness in hands or feet.

The 'deep' breathing exercises outlined below may help you to feel calmer and reduce some of the unpleasant bodily sensations. You could practise these exercises every day for five to ten minutes so that if you enter a situation that makes you feel very anxious you will be confident about using this technique.

Diaphragmatic breathing using the lower part of your lungs is one of the best ways to lower *stress* in the body. This is because when you *breathe* deeply, it sends a message to your brain to calm down and relax. The brain then sends this message to your body. The diaphragm is the most efficient muscle of breathing. It is a large, dome-shaped muscle located at the base of the lungs. Your abdominal muscles help move the diaphragm and give you more power to empty your lungs.

1. Sit comfortably, with your knees bent and your shoulders, head and neck relaxed.
2. Place one hand on your upper chest and the other just below your ribcage. This will allow you to feel your diaphragm move as you breathe.
3. Breathe in slowly through your nose so that your

stomach moves out against your hand. The hand on your chest should remain as still as possible.

4. Tighten your stomach muscles, letting them fall inwards as you exhale through tightly pressed (pursed) lips. The hand on your upper chest must remain as still as possible.

It can take a while to get this technique right. But keep at it, because with continued practice, diaphragmatic breathing will become easy and automatic. Once you can manage it sitting down, you will be able to use it wherever you please, be it on a train, standing in a queue or in a classroom.

Keep a record of your 'exposure tasks'

This will enable you to track your progress at facing 'challenging' situations. Over time you will hopefully notice a decrease in the level of your anxiety and be able to move on to the more difficult things on your list. Although the exposure record asks you to rate your anxiety level before, during and after each exposure task, it may be impractical to do so. Instead, you may want to make a note of your scores on a notepad or your phone and write them down on your record at a convenient time.

An example of a completed exposure task record of someone who felt anxious in social situations, and a blank one for you to photocopy, are given on pages 241–3.

Example of a completed exposure task record

Please record your activities and rate how 'anxious' you feel before, during and after each 'exposure' task, using the scale below.

0	1	2	3	4	5	6	7	8
No anxiety		Slight anxiety		Moderate anxiety		Marked anxiety		Severe anxiety/ distress

Date	Time Start/ Finish	Task	Before	During	After	Comments
15.06	9.30–10.30	Have one close friend round for coffee.	5	3	0	Went well, after initial anxiety.
18.06	10.30–11.00	Have two close friends over for coffee.	4	2	0	Felt less worried to start with. Enjoyed myself.
23.06	19:00–20.00	Meet two friends for a drink in the evening.	6	3	1	Felt flustered, couldn't park and was late. Then felt OK after a while. Need to get a street map!
01.07	12.00–14.00	Meet close friend and two friends I know less well for lunch.	3	2	0	Felt slightly nervous at first, but the girls I knew less well were really nice, so it worked out well.
07.07	1.30–3.00	Go to a friend's for a BBQ and meet new people.	2	1	0	Went well. Met some nice new people. Feeling more confident about starting college now.

Exposure task record

Please record your activities on the opposite page and rate how 'anxious' you feel before, during and after each 'exposure' task, using the scale below.

0	1	2	3	4	5	6	7	8
No anxiety stress		Slight anxiety		Moderate anxiety		Marked anxiety		Severe anxiety/ distress

Date	Time Start/ Finish	Task	Before	During	After	Comments

Points to bear in mind when tackling worries, stress and anxiety related to fatigue

- You may need to practise the techniques a few times to gain any benefit from them.
- You may need to use more than one of the techniques to overcome a particular worry or problem. For example, if one of your worries is whether or not to do a course, you may need to try problem solving to make a decision. Once you have made a decision you may need to do some exposure tasks to help you to overcome specific worries, such as meeting new people, travelling by yourself, etc.
- You can also use behavioural experiments as a way to test out your worries or fears, as discussed in Chapter 9.
- Remember to challenge any unhelpful thoughts that may occur along the way, as discussed in Chapter 9.
- Make sure that you plan a specific time to tackle your worries and write them down on your activity programme or target achievement record.

11

Overcoming blocks
to recovery

There may be times when you feel that although you are doing everything possible to help yourself to get better, you are having some problems in making progress. You may be following your programme conscientiously, but find that you are taking two steps forward and one step back. This can be extremely frustrating and can sometimes make you feel like doing things as and when you are able rather than following a consistent pattern of activity and rest, as recommended in this book.

It may be that you are being obstructed by one or more 'blocks'. These may be things of which you are totally unaware, or which you may sense in the back of your mind. If you can confront and deal with them, you will hopefully find it easier to make further progress.

This chapter presents a list of common blocks, with a few suggestions on how to tackle each of them, including notes on which parts of this book in particular may help you. We have left some space for you at the end of the chapter to add in any other blocks that you may notice, and room for you to write down your plans for how to tackle them.

Worry about increased activity making your symptoms worse

It is completely understandable that you would worry about increasing your level of activity when you are already feeling fatigued and possibly experiencing pain or other symptoms. Maybe you have increased some activities in the past and felt worse for doing so. Maybe you have received conflicting views on how you should manage your fatigue. Some people may have suggested that you should rest as much as possible, which might confuse you when you are trying to do more.

However, worry associated with activity can impede progress in overcoming your fatigue, for the following reasons:

- Worry about doing more can prevent you from taking the steps that help you to overcome fatigue.
- Temporary increases in pain or fatigue that may occur as a direct result of doing more can be misinterpreted as doing yourself harm, and this can then lead you to reduce the amount that you do rather than continue to attempt a gradual increase.

In order to overcome these difficulties, you may find it helpful to re-read the following sections of the book:

- Chapter 1 may help you to understand your symptoms better.
- Chapter 7 will tell you how to increase your levels of activity *gradually*. It will also reassure you that a slight increase in symptoms is normal when you change what you do, and that any such increase usually lasts only a short time.
- Chapter 9 may help you to challenge any 'worrying' thoughts you may have about your symptoms.

Recapping these chapters will help you to feel more confident about gradually increasing your levels of activity and accepting a temporary increase in symptoms.

Perfectionism

We have already discussed how, for some people, 'perfectionistic' personality traits may be one of the many contributory factors in chronic fatigue syndrome (see Figure 2.1, page 33). Having extremely high personal standards and expectations of yourself, and feeling distressed if you are unable to meet them, may also form a block to recovery, which may lead to problems like the ones listed below:

- trying to complete an activity in one go (e.g. writing an essay or painting a room) – this is likely to increase your feelings of exhaustion, which may then lead to you taking excessive rest);

- not being able to relax properly, as you feel you 'should' be doing something 'useful';
- avoiding new activities or not resuming previous activities for fear of not doing them well enough;
- finding it difficult to finish tasks because of excessive doubts that lead you to check things or do things repeatedly and make it difficult for you to move on to another task (e.g. when writing emails or an essay, or doing housework);
- never feeling that you have done anything well enough, which may make you feel dissatisfied;
- having an overly active 'inner critic', tending to focus on the things that you have not done and ignoring all that you have done.

If you can relate to some of the above problems, we suggest that you have another look at Chapter 9, as it will help you to understand how your perfectionistic thoughts may affect your symptoms, behaviour and emotions. You will then be guided on how to challenge your unhelpful thoughts and beliefs related to perfectionism that may be making your progress more difficult.

Other strategies that may also be helpful include the following:

- Write down three things that you have done each day, however small they might seem: e.g. did the washing-up, phoned a friend, did five minutes' reading, got out of bed on time.

- Praise yourself for things that you have done, rather than criticise yourself for things that you haven't done.
- Include pleasurable and fun activities in your day, rather than focus on things you feel you 'should' be doing.

For more ideas, read *Overcoming Perfectionism* by Roz Shafran, Sarah Egan and Tracey Wade in this series; 'Dare To Be Average', a chapter in *Feeling Good* by David Burns; and, 'Self-Bullying and How to Challenge It', a chapter in *Overcoming Depression* by Paul Gilbert, in this series. (For details see Chapter 14, 'Useful resources'.) There is also a useful website about self-compassion that can be very helpful for the 'self-critic':

www.compassionatemind.co.uk.

Receiving benefits or income protection

When you are severely restricted by your fatigue, there is no doubt that financial support, whether from the state or an insurance company, is very important. However, in certain situations it can make it difficult for you to make progress, for the following reasons.

- You may feel trapped by your benefits or policy if the conditions stipulate that you can work only for a few hours a week, can earn only a certain (small) amount a week, or may not do any work at all. Although you may feel that you have improved and are able to do *some* work, you may not want to endanger your financial support, fearing that if you come off benefit or relinquish your income protection you may then find that you cannot manage your work and face future financial problems.

- You may be having to attend regular medical check-ups or appeals; these can be very stressful and time-consuming and make it more difficult for you to concentrate on gradually increasing your activity levels.

- You may fear having to go back to a job that you feel contributed to you becoming ill in the first place.

If you feel that any of the above apply to your situation, you may find it helpful to read the information on 'Work, courses and resources in the UK' in Chapter 14 (pages 288–98). This will give you some information about benefits, income protection, employment, educational schemes and voluntary work. Although this information was up to date when the book was published, changes occur quite frequently, and therefore we would advise you to check on the relevant websites or discuss your situation with a Citizens Advice Bureau (CAB) adviser.

You may want to consider enrolling on a course or doing some voluntary work to build up your stamina and confidence gradually before going back to paid work. If you are worried about your financial position, it may be worth writing down your expenditure and income, with a view to appraising realistically how much leeway you have.

If you are receiving payments under an income protection policy (IP), a number of strategies may be helpful: for example, thinking about the advantages and disadvantages of being on IP. You may find it useful to do this with the aid of the problem-solving sheets on pages 231–4. You may wish to discuss different ways of returning to work with your employer or Occupational Health department if your place of employment has one. They may be more than happy for you to return to work in a graded way, starting with just a few hours a week, or you may discuss the possibility of returning to part-time work or doing some work from home.

Alternatively, if you feel that you do not want to return to your previous job or are unable to, you may consider discussing different settlement options with your employer, such as a redundancy package.

Work issues

If you are working, you may be encountering a number of problems. For example, you may find that you have too much work to do in too little time or have too many deadlines to meet. If this is the case, have a chat with your manager to see if you can reach a compromise. If you are struggling with the hours that you work, or having to travel in rush hour, again, see if there is any room for negotiation.

If you are considering going back to work, you may have some natural concerns about this. You may feel that your employer does not really understand your fatigue problems. If this is the case, you could photocopy some of the information from the book that you feel is relevant, for example Chapter 15 'Some guidelines for partners, relatives and friends'. If you are doing a graded return to work, you may be receiving some guidance and support from your Occupational Health department (if you have one). They may be suggesting a plan of how many hours you work and how to increase the hours over the next few weeks or months. If you do not have an Occupational Health department, you may need to negotiate your hours with your employer or manager. It is important to be realistic about how many hours you do to begin with to ensure that you are able to maintain your work. It would also be helpful for you to discuss taking breaks with your manager. You may find this difficult if you were not previously taking breaks; however, you will be more likely to be able to keep working if you take them. Depending on your job, could you schedule your breaks in your work diary or set a reminder on your phone? This may increase the likelihood that you take them. There may be somewhere at work where you can lie down or sit quietly for your break; again, have a word with your employer or manager.

For other work issues that we have not covered above, have a look at the section on problem solving on page 228, as this may help you to come up with some good alternatives to address your specific issue.

Other illness

Having another illness can be a considerable obstacle to consistent progress. You may have increased pain or other symptoms in addition to those associated with your fatigue that make it more difficult to stick to a structured activity programme or to sleep well. If your mood is depressed, this too can increase feelings of fatigue. If you get a lot of recurrent infections, for example of the chest or urinary tract, you are likely to feel even more unwell and may find it difficult to sleep and do your planned activities.

If your sleep is disturbed, you may like to re-read Chapter 6 on 'Improving your sleep'; this offers some strategies that may help you. You could also read Chapter 12 on 'Managing setbacks'. If you have an infection that comes and goes, this chapter will help you cope when your symptoms are more severe.

If you are under the care of another health-care professional for treatment of another condition, it may be helpful to tell them that you are trying to overcome your chronic fatigue using the cognitive behavioural strategies described in this book.

Conflicting advice or different kinds of therapy/diet

There is a lot of conflicting information about what is helpful in overcoming chronic fatigue or chronic fatigue syndrome. Although there is evidence to support cognitive behavioural therapy, some health professionals may suggest other treatments for which there is little or no evidence. This can be confusing.

Starting new treatments or diets for your fatigue while you are trying to follow the advice given in this book can make it more difficult for you to concentrate fully on your programme or to work out what is influencing improvements or changes in your symptoms. We would therefore recommend that you try just to stick to the recommendations given in this book. Also, if you avoid starting other treatments for your fatigue while you are working through this book, you will have a better idea about what has influenced improvement; this will equip you better to deal with any future recurrence of symptoms. In the unlikely circumstances that you notice a significant change or increase in your symptoms while working through this book, then we would suggest that you see your GP.

The 'wrong' kind of social support

This may sound like a contradiction! How could any social support be 'wrong'? However, certain kinds of support can make it more difficult for you to move forward. Occasionally, well-meaning friends or relatives may be concerned that your programme of planned activities and rest, and some of what it involves, will make your symptoms worse. They may base this view to some extent on past experience. Of course, they will have your best interests at heart, but may be too close to the problem to see it objectively.

If you find that those close to you have this kind of reservation about the programme you are following, try to reassure them that you believe this approach to be the right one, and that, although it takes time, there is evidence that it can help you to get better. You could also ask them to read the information for partners, relatives and friends in Chapter 15.

You may also consider photocopying the chapter for other people with whom you are in frequent contact, such as a tutor or an employer, to help them understand your fatigue problem. It may open up conversations about how they may be able to support you.

If you worry about telling people what you want or don't want, you might find it helpful to have a look again at the discussion of problem solving on pages 228–34, or to re-read the chapters on unhelpful thinking patterns. There are also some useful books on assertiveness.

A lack of social support

A lack of social support, forcing you to rely entirely on yourself, can make it difficult for you to make progress. If you live alone and have no family members or close friends nearby, you may find it hard to look after yourself properly in practical matters, for example cooking meals and doing the shopping. It may also be more difficult for you to persevere with your programme if you have a bad day and there is no one to offer you any support or encouragement.

If this situation applies to you and you are greatly restricted by your illness, it may be helpful to consider talking to your

GP, who may be able to organise an assessment of your situation with a view to some practical support. It may also be useful to talk to neighbours to see if they could help you occasionally. There may be small things that you can do for them in return. You might ask friends who live a little way away whether they could call in from time to time.

Cultural issues

Religious and cultural beliefs can affect the way we react to and think about illness. The illness may be perceived as a 'test from God' or a punishment for wrongdoing. You may feel, or be told by others, that if your faith was strong enough you would be able to overcome your illness. You may even feel guilty for not being grateful for all that you do have. Some cultures believe that illness and bad luck can be caused by others who want to harm you via supernatural sources. You might be advised to seek a 'traditional healer' to fix the problem.

Turning to faith in times of need is understandable. It is a source of hope and strength for many and it sometimes helps make sense of why bad things happen. However, it is equally important to make use of all the help that is available.

Some cultures have difficulty in accepting certain kinds of illness, particularly if an obvious physical cause cannot be found. If this applies to you, or to those close to you, it may result in you continuing to have many unnecessary tests rather than concentrating on your CBT programme. Just because an organic cause for your fatigue cannot be found, this does not mean the physical symptoms you are experiencing are not real. You may find it helpful to review Chapter 1 for a detailed explanation of symptoms. Relatives and friends may find the information in Chapter 15 helpful.

Ongoing 'stressful' situations

Stress of any sort can make it more difficult for you to make consistent progress, however hard you try. Stress can increase your levels of fatigue and other symptoms, and can also make it more difficult for you to 'switch off' at bedtime or when you are supposed to be resting or relaxing.

Potentially stressful situations include the following:

- Life events, whether good, bad or neutral, such as moving house, getting married, starting a new job or a bereavement.
- Financial difficulties that may have occurred as a result of not being able to work or doing less work.
- Environment: you may live in an uncomfortable, unpleasant or chaotic environment where it may be difficult to relax. You may feel that your home is in a mess, as you have difficulty keeping it tidy or clean. There may be a lot of noise in your home or nearby, perhaps from other occupants, neighbours or traffic. Your house may be too hot or too cold. You may not get on with the people with whom you live.
- Relationship difficulties, with your partner or other family members.

- Loneliness, maybe because you live alone or because you have lost friends or cannot go out very often because of your fatigue.
- Illness of a family member or other problems within the family.

If any of the above situations apply to you, you might find reading Chapter 10 on 'Overcoming worry, stress and anxiety related to your chronic fatigue' helpful. The section on problem solving may help you to think about alternative ways of tackling your situation. You may also want to think about planning a short daily time specifically for thinking about how to address your problems: for more information, see the section titled 'Problem-solving strategy for reducing worries at night' on pages 99–101. Don't forget to set aside time to relax. Discussing worries with a close friend or relative (if appropriate) may be helpful. Finally, make use of any available resources relevant to your particular problem: for example, financial advisers or your bank to discuss financial issues, landlords/environmental health department to discuss problematic living conditions.

Breaking through comfort zones

If you have had fatigue for a long time, you may have stopped doing a lot of things that you used to do. Some may be big parts of your life, such as working, socialising or studying. Others may be quite small things, such as paying bills or phoning people. Whenever any of us stop doing things for some time, we lose confidence in our ability to do them. It may be that a lack of confidence in your ability to do things, or worry about things not going according to plan, is stopping you from resuming your former activities.

Again, if you feel that any of this applies to you, you may find it helpful to read Chapter 10 on 'Overcoming worry, stress and anxiety related to your chronic fatigue', which describes some strategies that will help you to resume old activities and try new ones. In addition, Chapter 9, 'Overcoming unhelpful thinking patterns', may offer some useful hints.

Finally, write a list of things that you have not done for a long time and would like to do, and put them in order from easy to difficult. Incorporate one or two items from your list into your programme each week.

On the next page, you will find space to note down your own particular block(s), with room beneath to note down your plans.

My own blocks (s)

1.

•
_____
_____
_____
_____

2.

•
_____
_____
_____
_____

3.

•
_____
_____
_____
_____

4.

•
_____
_____
_____
_____

12

Managing setbacks

There may be times when you have a setback: that is, an increase in symptoms for more than a few days. Although this may seem really difficult at the time, it can help you to gain a better understanding of your fatigue problem and enhance the way that you manage it in the future. Most people overcome their setbacks quite easily and go on to make further progress. The important thing is not to panic!

A setback may occur when you are working through this book, or after you have finished. If you have a setback, you may feel that you are sliding backwards and that, instead of maintaining your levels of activity, you are returning to old patterns: for example, resting in response to symptoms, sleeping in the day, or overdoing it when you have a bit of energy. You may feel despondent and be uncertain what to do for the best.

It is important to understand that a setback cannot always be avoided, but it can be dealt with quite easily. The key is to be able to recognise a setback if it occurs, and to tackle it by taking some positive action.

Common triggers of setbacks

Setbacks usually occur for a reason, although it can sometimes be challenging to work out what it is. There are times when they are more likely to occur. The situations listed below can increase fatigue and make it more difficult for you to continue regular planned activities and relaxation.

- Getting an infection or another illness.
- Experiencing any major life event e.g. moving house, a bereavement, changing jobs, getting married or divorced.
- Stressful conditions: e.g. if you have builders/decorators working at your home, you have deadlines to meet at work or college, or you are experiencing relationship issues or family problems.
- Depressed mood.
- Ceasing to use the techniques described in this book and resuming old patterns of behaviour.

How to tackle setbacks

Listed below are a variety of strategies to help you tackle your setback and get back on track.

- If you have a temperature or another illness on top of your chronic fatigue, it is important that you increase your rest for a day or so until your temperature returns to normal.

- Do *not* be tempted to increase your rest periods for too long, or until all of your symptoms subside, as this may prolong your recovery.
- Try to nip your problems in the bud as soon as you realise that you are not managing so well with your programme, as it will then take you less time to get back on track.
- Prioritise your activities if you do not have time to or do not feel able to carry out all your programme. You could use 'problem solving' to help you with this.
- Remember to balance your days as much as possible in terms of a variety of activities and relaxation.
- Lower your expectations of what you can manage and praise yourself for your achievements.
- Discuss your concerns with a family member or a friend and maybe ask them for some help or support.
- If your fatigue or any other symptoms remain increased for more than a few weeks, then make an appointment to see your doctor.

What if I have a setback after finishing working through the book?

- Go back to basics. Review all of the information in the book, but initially focus on Chapter 6 ('Improving your sleep') and Chapter 7 ('Planning activity and rest').
- It may be worth keeping an activity diary and a sleep diary (if sleep is a problem) for a week, to identify your patterns of activity, rest and sleep.

- Using the information in your activity diary and sleep diary, construct a basic activity programme to tackle the problem areas.
- Ensure that you plan manageable chunks of a variety of activities, with regular relaxation/rest periods.
- To monitor your progress, you may like to continue to record your activities in an activity diary or on a target achievement record until you feel a little better.
- If you continue to have problems overcoming a setback after trying these methods for a few weeks, make an appointment with your doctor.
- Refer to the information above about 'how to tackle setbacks' and write your setback plan on page 286.

PART THREE

MAKING FURTHER PROGRESS

Introduction

We hope that by the time you reach this part of the book, you will not only have found some useful ways of managing your chronic fatigue but be feeling better and on your way to recovery.

This section aims to help you to evaluate your progress, identify any remaining problems and learn how to consolidate your gains and make further progress.

We suggest that you start working through this part of the book once you have worked through all the chapters that are relevant to you, when you are feeling a little better and are well on your way to achieving some of your targets. In reality, this may take a few months

First, we thought that you might like to hear an update about Sarah, Alison and Ben, who we introduced in Chapter 2. They all used strategies described in the book alongside sessions of CBT.

Sarah

Sarah attended sessions over seven months and then four follow-ups at three-monthly intervals over the next year.

You will have seen some of the examples of her diaries and work that she did throughout the book. By session fourteen, she was feeling fatigued for about 50 per cent of the time but felt it was more manageable. She was going out socially and exercising more often. She had completed her second year at university and was generally feeling more confident, happier in her mood and less anxious. At her three-month follow-up, her fatigue had reduced further, and she felt that it was not really stopping her from doing anything. At her six-month follow-up, she reported that she had had a slight increase in her fatigue at the beginning of her third year at university. Despite not being able to attend all of her lectures, she was liaising with her tutors and keeping on top of her work at home. She was making a supreme effort to continue to see her friends and enter social situations that she would have previously found difficult due to anxiety. At her final follow-up, she had completed her degree and was thinking about her work options. She was considering starting with some part-time voluntary work to build her confidence and stamina before finding paid work. She was keeping up with walking daily and had been for her first short run. Her mood and anxiety remained improved.

Alison

Alison attended fortnightly sessions over about eight months and then three follow-up sessions over the next year. By the end of her regular sessions, she had managed to increase her walks further and was resting for only three hours a day as opposed to between six and eight hours at the beginning of her sessions. She was seeing friends more regularly, doing more of the housework and shopping, and had registered for a creative writing course. Her relationship with her husband had improved, as he had a better understanding of her CFS and was not having to do all of the chores. At her three-month follow-up, she had started a creative writing course and was really enjoying it. She was able to do more with her son, such as go to the park with him, have his friends round for meals and help him with his homework. Her progress had continued at her six-month follow-up and she had taken over most of the things that she had stopped doing at home. She reported at her one-year follow-up that she had returned to part-time work at the nursery school.

Overall, Alison felt that CBT strategies outlined in the book had improved her understanding of CFS and had equipped her with some useful ways to tackle the problems associated with it. She decided that she did not want to return to full-time work, as she was enjoying having some free time and wanted to do some further courses. Her confidence in her ability to get on with people had greatly improved and she had made some new friendships as well as resuming some old ones.

Ben

Made steady progress over his course of sessions. His main targets were to work full time and run long distances again.

At the end of treatment, he had started a full-time job as an accounts assistant and was managing this well. He had built up his running to twenty-six miles over three days a week. He was sleeping well, felt positive in his mood and no longer felt that he had a problem with fatigue. At his three-month, six-month and nine-month follow-up, all was continuing to go well. He started a sports therapy B-Tech course in which he was attending weekend lectures. He therefore decided to reduce his working days to four. He continued to gradually build up his running and to run in competitive races.

By his nine-month follow-up, he was running up to sixty miles per week and had plans for a prestigious competitive race the following month. He also had other running goals, including a marathon the following year. He felt that he had totally recovered. We discussed what he felt had been key to his recovery. There were various points he raised that he was happy for me to share with you:

Acceptance – that it would take time to get better. Also, in order to get better, he needed to reduce his exercise and stop work for a while.

Diet – having a healthy balanced diet and eating at regular times.

Having a regular getting-up and going-to-bed time.

Planned activities and breaks throughout the day.

Gradually increasing activity.

Taking a step back when things were more difficult and rationalising his unhelpful thoughts.

Being mindful of what he had been through in terms of being unwell, and not allowing himself to get too carried away when feeling better.

He also felt that his illness had allowed him to look at his life differently and to think about what his priorities were, including things that made him happy. He concluded that money wasn't everything and therefore decided to focus more on his love of sport than having a well-paid job.

13

Preparing for the future

Well done for reaching this part of the book! We hope that by now you will be feeling more confident about managing your chronic fatigue, be feeling a little better and be doing more of what you want to do. In this chapter, we discuss how to sustain your improvement and to build on your progress. We also help you to think about triggers for setbacks so that you are prepared to nip those problems in the bud should they arise.

How do I sustain my improvements?

There may be so many things that you have done to get to this point in the book and that have contributed to your improvement. Some may be fairly straightforward, such as having a good routine in the day with a regular getting-up time, planned breaks or rests and a variety of planned activities. However, you may have made other changes that have helped you, such as connecting with friends again, asking for help, delegating tasks to others, reducing your high standards to reduce the pressure you put on yourself.

It is useful to take time to consider what you feel has helped you, so that you can ensure that you keep those particular things going. We have included an 'Evaluation of progress' form on pages 281–2 to help you to do this.

The following suggestions aim to help you to sustain the improvements that you have made and build on your progress:

- Continue with your activity programme in terms of keeping up with a structured routine of planned activity and rest. You may have reduced your rests as you have gradually felt better; this is entirely appropriate. However, do not be tempted just to stop or miss out rests, as this may result in you sliding backwards.

- Make sure that your lifestyle is balanced between a mixture of different kinds of activity and relaxation.

- Include at least half an hour to one hour for yourself each day to do exactly what you *want* to do. This does not mean catching up on things you feel you should be doing!

- Ensure that you have regular short breaks when you are working, studying or looking after children, even if you do not feel that you have time or feel that you need them.

- Try to maintain a regular sleep pattern. If you are feeling better, you may not have to be as rigid with your getting-up times or going-to-bed times. It is fine to go to bed or get up a little later at times, so long as you do not find that it is too disruptive or that you start to have difficulty in getting to sleep or waking in the morning.

- Aim to do some exercise at least five days a week. What you do will depend on your own personal goals. However, walking even for a few minutes every day will be helpful.
- Eat regular meals.
- Prioritise your activities, ask for help or delegate if you find you have too much to do.
- Do make sure that you continue with the more subtle parts of your programme, such as core belief work, conducting behavioural experiments, as well as changes that you've made, such as expressing your needs, asking for help, prioritising yourself, etc.

How do I monitor and track my progress?

You may have been keeping records for a few months. Initially you may have been completing sleep and activity diaries, and then you may have moved on to target achievement records. In order to track your progress, you may find it helpful to continue to keep some sort of diary or record. It is not necessary for you to continue to complete activity diaries or target achievement records unless you find them particularly helpful. We have devised a record that tracks your progress and requires less writing. We have called this a 'Record of progress' and have provided two examples of completed records, followed by a blank one for you to photocopy, on pages 278–80.

You can continue with this as long as you find it to be helpful.

The idea of this record is to prioritise what you want to focus on. You may find it helpful to set aside a few minutes every week to begin with, to review how you've got on in the previous week. You do not need to write down all of your programme for the week, such as to swim weekly, do admin for an hour twice weekly, take three half-hour breaks daily, etc. but instead can choose a specific priority, such as: make time for myself to do what I want for an hour a day, to start looking for voluntary work, to get in touch with old friends. It will really help you to keep on track if you keep a regular review of your progress, as you are more likely to notice if things start to slide; you can then take some early action.

How do I make changes to my lifestyle?

Making changes is an important part of sustaining a lasting improvement. You may well have some targets that you are continuing to work towards and, if not, then you may consider setting yourself some new ones.

If you have been fatigued for a long time, not only may you have given up doing many things, such as working and socialising, but other people may have taken over some of your previous responsibilities, for example, shopping, cooking, paying bills, household repairs. If this is the case, you may decide that resuming some of these activities would be a positive step. Remember to take things gradually and, if necessary, to break them down into manageable steps and, of course, ask for help.

Evaluating progress

As we mentioned earlier in this chapter, it can be helpful to spend some time thinking about what you've found helpful from working through this book and what you need to continue to work on in order to make further progress. We recommend that you put half an hour or so aside at a convenient time to complete the 'Evaluation of progress' form on pages 281–2.

Working towards current or new targets

We have included three forms called 'Targets for the next three months'. You can use these forms to write down your targets at three-monthly intervals and to make a plan of how you will work towards them. You can change your time frame for your targets if you so wish. These forms can be found on pages 283–5.

Record of progress, example 1

Week beginning................

Date	Programme (List activities that I plan for the week.)	Comments (How did I get on with my programme?)	Plan (What can I do differently next week/fortnight?)
4th Sept.	Get up and get dressed by 9 a.m.	Did very well with getting up and going to bed on time.	Get up at 8.45 a.m. daily.
	Have three one-hour rests.	Rested a bit longer than one hour each time.	Set an alarm clock to make sure that I get up from my rest on time.
	Go for two fifteen-minute walks daily.	Didn't manage two walks each day.	Try to do the walks at regular times e.g. 10 a.m. and 6 p.m.
	Read for half an hour, twice daily.	Managed planned reading.	Increase the reading to 40 minutes twice daily.
	Meet a friend for lunch for one hour weekly.	Met friend weekly.	Meet a friend twice weekly for up to one and a half hours.
	Go to bed by 11 p.m.	Generally, did well.	Keep bedtime the same.

Record of progress, example 2

Week beginning................

Date	Programme (List activities that I plan for the week.)	Comments (How did I get on with my programme?)	Plan (What can I do differently next week/fortnight?)
4th Sept.	1. Try to get back into the routine of going to the gym again on a regular basis. Go to the gym 3 × for ½ hour each week.	Managed to go to gym three times during the first week and twice in the second week.	Did pretty well with my gym attendance. I will try to keep it up during the next fortnight.
	2. Go out with friends to celebrate birthday; be home by midnight to avoid too much fatigue following day.	Had a good night out but didn't manage to get home until really late. Felt really awful the next day and therefore didn't go to the gym.	Try harder to get home by midnight when I go out to a concert this week, so that I don't miss out on other enjoyable things the day after.
	3. Hunt for new flat.	Found this really exhausting, but managed to find a new flat.	Try to ensure that I have some planned relaxation time of at least 1 hour a day as I am conscious that this is slipping.

279

Record of progress

Week beginning.................................

Date	Programme (List activities that I plan for the week.)	Comments (How did I get on with my programme?)	Plan (What can I do differently next week/fortnight?)

Managing setbacks

You will have already read about how to manage a setback in Chapter 12. In order to try to prevent setbacks, or minimise them if they occur, it is helpful to think about your own triggers of setbacks, and the strategies that you could implement to deal with them. We have therefore devised a 'Preventing setbacks' form for you to complete; this can be found on page 286.

EVALUATION OF PROGRESS

Please complete the following sections in as much detail as possible.

1(a) *What are the main things I have learned about CFS/my fatigue problem?*

_____

_____

_____

_____

1(b) *What factors may have preceded my CFS/fatigue problem?*
(E.g. constantly being busy, recurrent infections, aiming for perfection.)

_____

_____

_____

_____

1(c) *What factors may have contributed to my fatigue continuing?*
(E.g. an erratic sleep pattern, long periods of activity followed by
long rests, taking too much on.)

_____

_____

_____

_____

2 *What strategies have I found helpful while working through this book?*
(E.g. having regular breaks, going to bed at a set time, challenging
unhelpful thoughts, changing expectations of myself.)

_____

_____

_____

_____

3 *What areas do I still need to work on to make further progress?*
(E.g. targets I have not yet achieved, resting at regular times, work
on core beliefs.)

_____

_____

_____

_____

Now please turn to the next page to think about what you would
like to work towards in the next three months.

TARGETS FOR THE NEXT THREE MONTHS

Please write down targets that you plan to work towards during the next three months.

_____

_____

_____

_____

_____

_____

_____

_____

Write a detailed plan of how you aim to work towards each of your targets.

_____

_____

_____

_____

_____

_____

_____

_____

Evaluate your progress at the end of three months and then turn to the next page to plan your targets for the next three months.

TARGETS FOR THE NEXT THREE MONTHS

Please write down targets that you plan to work towards during the next three months.

_____

_____

_____

_____

_____

_____

_____

_____

Write a detailed plan of how you aim to work towards each of your targets.

_____

_____

_____

_____

_____

_____

_____

_____

Evaluate your progress at the end of three months and then turn to the next page to plan your targets for the next three months.

TARGETS FOR THE NEXT THREE MONTHS

Please write down targets that you plan to work towards during the next three months.

_____

_____

_____

_____

_____

_____

_____

_____

Write a detailed plan of how you aim to work towards each of your targets.

_____

_____

_____

_____

_____

_____

_____

_____

PREVENTING SETBACKS

Review the information in Chapter 11 on 'Managing setbacks' to help you to complete this sheet.

Can I identify any warning signs or triggers that make my fatigue worse? (E.g. when I am very busy/get an infection, don't sleep well, have more difficulty getting out of bed.)

_____

_____

_____

_____

_____

_____

_____

_____

What steps do I need to take if I find myself getting into difficulties? (E.g. ensure that I take planned breaks and slightly increase them, if necessary, do not stay in bed all day, discuss with a partner or friend, ask for help, prioritise my activities.)

_____

_____

_____

_____

_____

_____

_____

14

Useful resources

In this chapter we provide details of a number of resources that we hope will help you to make further progress. These include useful books, contacts to help in finding work and educational opportunities, information on benefits and where to get advice and suggestions on how to find specialist help and therapy. For information and professional help in countries other than the UK, please see the Appendix.

Further reading

Many of the books listed below give very good practical advice in overcoming a number of problems that we have not been able to include in much detail.

David D. Burns, *Feeling Good* (Avon Books, 1999)

Melanie Fennell, *Overcoming Low Self-esteem*, 2nd edition: *A self-help guide using cognitive behavioural techniques* (Robinson, 2016)

Paul Gilbert, *Overcoming Depression*, 3rd edition: *A self-help guide using cognitive behavioural techniques* (Robinson, 2009)

Dennis Greenberger and Christine Padesky, *Mind over Mood*, 2nd edition (Guilford Press, 2015)

Helen Kennerley, *Overcoming Anxiety*, 2nd edition: *A self-help guide using cognitive behavioural techniques* (Robinson, 2014)

Work, courses and resources in the UK

If you are considering returning to work, doing a course, or finding a new job, it can be difficult to know where to start. You may be aware of your entitlements, opportunities available to you and where to go for help. On the other hand, you may not be, in which case we hope that the information below is of help to you. Please note that the information was correct at the time of publication.

Equality Act 2010

What is it?

The Equality Act 2010 legally protects people from discrimination in the workplace and in wider society.

It replaced previous anti-discrimination laws with a single Act, making the law easier to understand and strengthening protection in some situations. It sets out the different ways in which it's unlawful to treat someone.

The Equality Act 2010 prohibits discrimination against people with the protected characteristics that are specified in section 4 of the Act. Disability is one of the specified protected characteristics. Protection from discrimination for disabled people applies to disabled people in a range of circumstances, covering the provision of goods, facilities and services, the exercise of public functions, premises, work, education and associations. Only those disabled people who are defined as disabled in accordance with section 6 of the Act, and the associated schedules and regulations made under that section, will be entitled to the protection that the Act provides to disabled people. However, the Act also provides protection for non-disabled people who are subjected to direct discrimination or harassment because of their association with a disabled person or because they are wrongly perceived to be disabled.

Definition of disability

The Act defines a disabled person as a person with a disability. You're disabled under the Equality Act 2010 if you have a physical or mental impairment that has a 'substantial' and 'long-term' negative effect on your ability to do normal daily activities.

Included

A disability can arise from a wide range of impairments that can be:

- Sensory impairments, such as those affecting sight or hearing.

- Impairments with fluctuating or recurring effects such as rheumatoid arthritis, myalgic encephalitis (ME), chronic fatigue syndrome, fibromyalgia, depression and epilepsy.
- Progressive conditions, such as motor neurone disease, muscular dystrophy and forms of dementia.
- Auto-immune conditions such as systemic lupus erythematosus (SLE).
- Organ-specific, including respiratory conditions, such as asthma, and cardiovascular diseases, including thrombosis, stroke and heart disease.
- Developmental, such as autistic spectrum disorders (ASD), dyslexia and dyspraxia.
- Learning disabilities.
- Mental health conditions with symptoms such as anxiety, low mood, panic attacks, phobias, or unshared perceptions; eating disorders; bipolar affective disorders; obsessive compulsive disorders; personality disorders; post-traumatic stress disorder; and some self-harming behaviour.
- Mental illnesses, such as depression and schizophrenia.
- Impairments due to injury to the body or brain.
  - It may not be possible, nor necessary, to categorise a condition as either a physical or mental impairment.
  - Not necessary to consider how an impairment is caused.
  - Account should be taken of how far a person can reasonably be expected to modify his or

her behaviour, for example by use of a coping or avoidance strategy, to prevent or reduce the effects of an impairment on normal day-to-day activities. In some instances, a coping or avoidance strategy might alter the effects of the impairment to the extent that they are no longer substantial, and the person would no longer meet the definition of disability.

What protection does it provide?

It is against the law for employers to discriminate against you because of a disability. The Equality Act 2010 protects you and covers areas including:

- Application forms.
- Interview arrangements.
- Aptitude or proficiency tests.
- Job offers.
- Terms of employment, including pay.
- Promotion, transfer and training opportunities.
- Dismissal or redundancy.
- Discipline and grievances.

An employer has to make 'reasonable adjustments' to avoid you being put at a disadvantage compared to non-disabled people in the workplace. For example, adjusting your working hours or providing you with a special piece of equipment to help you do the job.

An employer who's recruiting staff may make limited enquiries about your health or disability.

You can only be asked about your health or disability:

- To help decide if you can carry out a task that is an essential part of the work.
- To help find out if you can take part in an interview.
- To help decide if the interviewers need to make reasonable adjustments for you in a selection process.
- To help monitoring.
- If they want to increase the number of disabled people they employ.
- If they need to know for the purposes of national security checks.

You may be asked whether you have a health condition or disability on an application form or in an interview. You need to think about whether the question is one that is allowed to be asked at that stage of recruitment.

You can't be chosen for redundancy just because you're disabled. The selection process for redundancy must be fair and balanced for all employees.

Your employer cannot force you to retire if you become disabled.

Overview of protection

The Equality Act 2010 protects you from discrimination. It provides legal rights for you in the areas of:

- Employment.
- Education.
- Access to goods, services and facilities.
- Buying and renting land or property.

The Equality Act 2010 also protects your rights if you have an association with a disabled person, for example a carer or parent.

Under the Act, there is a range of services, concessions, schemes and financial benefits for which disabled people may qualify. These include, for example: local authority services for disabled people; the Blue Badge parking scheme; tax concessions for people who are blind; and disability-related social security benefits. However, each of these has its own individual eligibility criteria and qualification, for any one of them does not automatically confer entitlement to protection under the Act, nor does entitlement to the protection of the Act confer eligibility for benefits, or concessions. Please see the following websites for further information:

https://www.gov.uk/government/uploads/system/uploads/attachment_data/file/570382/Equality_Act_2010-disability_definition.pdf

https://www.gov.uk/rights-disabled-person/overview

Information for people who are receiving benefits

If you have been ill for some time, you may be receiving welfare benefits. Understandably, you may have concerns about how your income will be affected if you return to work. You may feel that you are ready for some part-time work, but are unsure about the financial implications.

The websites listed below may help you to find out more information about your entitlements.

https://www.gov.uk/incapacity-benefit

https://www.gov.uk/employment-support-allowance/overview

https://www.gov.uk/attendance-allowance/overview

https://www.gov.uk/carers-allowance/overview

https://www.gov.uk/working-tax-credit/overview

Income Protection (IP)

IP is a UK insurance scheme whereby you are paid an amount equivalent to part of your salary while you are unable to work. Usually, the policy is held between the employer and the insurance company. Many insurance companies are willing to negotiate a gradual return to work with part payment until full-time work is achieved. Some insurers are willing to pay for rehabilitation and cognitive behavioural therapy as a way of helping people to return to work. Some employers will offer redundancy packages on health grounds.

Income Protection policies are also available for the self-employed; under these, the insurance company makes regular payments (specified in the policy) if you are unable to pursue your usual work after an initial period of typically one to three months.

Employment and educational schemes

Below are a couple of UK-based websites through which you could find out information and advice on returning to work, finding new work (voluntary or paid), or doing a training or educational course:

http://www. jobcentreplus.gov.uk/JCP/index.html

Read more about staying safe online at safer-jobs.com https://www.gov.uk/jobsearch

Learndirect courses and centres

Learndirect offer a selection of Access to Higher Education Diplomas as well as other professional development courses and qualifications. You can do the majority of your studying remotely. In this way you can study around your existing commitments.

There are a variety of courses in a number of subject areas. Every course is also eligible for government-backed funding.

http://www.learndirect.com/.

Citizens Advice Bureau (CAB)

The Citizens Advice Bureau is an organisation that gives free, confidential, impartial and independent advice on a wide range of subjects, including employment, benefits, housing and debt.

For further information contact your nearest CAB by telephoning or dropping in during working hours, Monday to Friday. The CAB main website can be visited at https://www.citizensadvice.org.uk/.

Voluntary work

There are a variety of organisations that may be contacted with a view to finding out about doing voluntary work. Volunteering opportunities come in many shapes and sizes. Some people volunteer for a few hours regularly, others when called upon by an organisation. You could volunteer in your neighbourhood, online or in other countries.

Do-it

The UK's national volunteering database, Do-it.org, makes it easy for anyone to volunteer in their community.

Do-it.org lists over a million volunteering opportunities that are posted by volunteer centres, national/local charities and voluntary groups. Do-it ensures that almost 50,000 organisations find the help they need to provide vital services to the community.

Do-it.org was acquired from YouthNet in 2013. After redeveloping the service, Do-it was transferred to Vivo as part of the Trust's joint social enterprise partnership, Vivo Life, in 2017.

https://www.do-ittrust.org.

National Trust

The National Trust is an organisation that looks after a variety of buildings, including houses, gardens, coastline and countryside. There are many volunteering opportunities in areas throughout Great Britain.

https://www.nationaltrust.org.uk/volunteer.

NCVO

The National Council for Voluntary Organisations (NCVO) is the umbrella body for the voluntary sector in England.

https://www.ncvo.org.uk/ncvo-volunteering.

Website for information on CFS

The Persistent Physical Symptoms Research and Treatment Unit based at King's College Hospital, London, has a website offering further information about CFS:

https://www.national.slam.nhs.uk/services/adult-services/persistentphysicalsymptomsresearchandtreatmentunit.

Referral to a specialist

If you have found that this book has helped you, but feel that you would like to be seen by a specialist in chronic fatigue, ask your doctor if there is a specialist centre in your area and if you can be referred to it.

Finding a therapist

If, after working through this book, you would like to have some sessions of cognitive behavioural therapy with a therapist, you can ask your doctor to refer you to a qualified therapist in your area who specialises in working with people with fatigue. Alternatively, you can contact the British Association for Behavioural and Cognitive Psychotherapists (BABCP), which holds a list of accredited therapists who work both privately and in the NHS. You can contact it via the website https://www.babcp.com.

PART FOUR

HOW OTHERS CAN HELP

Introduction

This part of the book has some brief information for people who are close to you. It talks about what chronic fatigue syndrome is, and what may have contributed to its onset and be keeping it going. It also offers some suggestions about how others can help you. We hope that this section will be helpful to people close to you, whatever the cause of your fatigue.

15

Some guidelines for partners, relatives and friends

It can be extremely helpful to people suffering from fatigue, for whatever reason, to have someone who understands a little about their problems and the way in which they are trying to tackle them. The first part of this chapter gives some basic facts about chronic fatigue syndrome that will not apply to everyone. The second part guides you on helping them.

The purpose of this chapter is to give you:

- some basic facts about chronic fatigue syndrome;
- guidance on how you can help them to get the best out of this book.

Facts about chronic fatigue syndrome

What is chronic fatigue syndrome?

Chronic fatigue syndrome, also known as post-viral fatigue syndrome or myalgic encephalomyelitis (ME), is a condition that affects people in different ways. The main symptom is persistent fatigue, which can be severe and disabling, leading to a substantially restricted lifestyle. Other associated problems may include painful muscles and/or joints, sore throats, headaches, dizziness, poor concentration and memory loss. Problems with sleep are common: for example, sleeping more during the day, having difficulty in going to sleep at night and waking frequently. Sleep is seldom refreshing.

Symptoms and the consequences of them differ greatly among individuals. Approximately 25 per cent of people with CFS are housebound due to the severity of their symptoms. Other people may be able to carry out activities such as going to work or be able to look after the home and their children or do a course of study. However, the effort required to do these things may result in little energy to do other activities, such as seeing friends, exercising or other personal interests.

What causes CFS?

There has been a lot of speculation about different causes of CFS, but it is unlikely that a single cause will ever be identified. However, a combination of some of the following factors seems to be associated with the onset of the illness in many cases:

- an initial illness or a series of infections;
- leading a busy or stressful lifestyle, whether at work or at home;

- stressful life events such as bereavement, moving house, changing jobs, getting married, ending a long-term relationship: all these may lead to increased vulnerability to infections and/or fatigue;
- having high personal expectations and striving to do things 'perfectly': this can be stressful and at times, exhausting.

What keeps CFS going?

People often wonder why CFS keeps on going, months or maybe years after the person first became ill. Some of the reasons are listed below.

- Resuming previous activities, e.g., working too soon after an initial infection may delay recovery.
- Resting too much once an initial infection or illness has subsided can cause the body to become out of condition; this in turn can particularly adversely affect the muscles, immune system and nervous system. Problems that may follow include an increased proneness to illness, and symptoms including muscle weakness and feeling sluggish, with poor memory and poor concentration.
- Alternating over-vigorous activity or exercise with resting for long periods can inadvertently make fatigue worse in the longer term, as the body does not get used to a consistent pattern of activity and rest.

- An irregular bedtime or getting-up time, or resting or sleeping too much in the day, may contribute to disturbed and unrefreshing sleep at night. Not sleeping well at night is likely to increase feelings of fatigue and other symptoms.

- Worries about symptoms may lead people to stop or reduce certain activities. This restriction of lifestyle in turn can cause them to feel frustrated and demoralised, which in turn can adversely affect symptoms.

- Receiving advice from a variety of sources can lead to confusion and uncertainty about what to do for the best.

- The debilitating effects of CFS can lead to significant problems and life changes, e.g. financial difficulties, reduced social contacts, or changing roles within the family. These difficulties can understandably trigger feelings such as frustration and helplessness. These feelings, which are a natural human response to stress, can then lead to low mood for some people. Low mood itself can lead to problems including tiredness, which can exacerbate fatigue and further reduce the desire to be active.

How can you help?

If you are close to someone with CFS or fatigue associated with another illness who is using this book, your understanding and support can be extremely helpful in assisting them to get better. This book describes a variety of techniques based on cognitive behavioural therapy (CBT). This is a pragmatic approach that is helpful to people with a variety of illnesses. Some people with CFS, as well as fatigue that occurs for other reasons, can find CBT beneficial.

The following are some ways in which you may be able to help your partner, relative or friend.

- Discuss with the person their views on how they best feel that you can help them. It may be that they want you to be significantly involved e.g. by accompanying them on planned walks, phoning them to make sure they are out of bed, or discussing their progress on a daily basis. On the other hand, they may want to get on with their programme by themselves but want just a little bit of support and encouragement from you.
- Take time to read the information in this chapter so that you understand a little more about CFS and what they are trying to do to overcome it. You may also find it helpful to read some of the chapters for more detailed information.
- If you are aware of targets they are working on as part of their activity programme, give praise for anything they achieve. Your encouragement will help them to recognise that they are making progress. Achievements may seem very small – for example, getting up fifteen minutes earlier each day, walking for a minute further each day, not sleeping during the day – but they often require huge amounts of effort.

- Encourage all efforts that the person is making in relation to their programme, whether it is doing a particular homework activity, filling in their activity diaries, or reading information in this book. The techniques described in this book are time-consuming and require a lot of effort, so the more support anyone gets in using them the better. Remind them that they are likely to feel better if they persevere with their programme and that small step-by-step achievements are the key to success.

- When your partner/relative/friend starts to tackle their unhelpful thoughts, they will initially be trying to identify thoughts that may be hampering their progress, such as 'I will never get better' or 'I should be able to do more'. Once the person can identify their unhelpful thoughts, they will learn to challenge them and try to think of more 'helpful' alternative thoughts. You may be asked to point out when they say something 'negative' or 'unhelpful'. Challenging unhelpful thoughts can be difficult, as it is not always easy to see a helpful alternative. This particularly applies when someone is feeling poorly, upset, worried or a bit low. If they are struggling, especially if progress is slow, you may be able to help by pointing out some helpful alternatives e.g. what they have achieved so far. You can refer to the questions on page 159 to give you some ideas.

Please also consider the following points:

- When starting to work through this book, the person may notice an increase in their symptoms. This is usually temporary and occurs as a result of changing their patterns of activity and rest. Encouragement and support at this time are particularly necessary, as they may feel like reducing their activities in response to an increase in symptoms. It is important to stress that any slight increase in symptoms is both normal and temporary, and that occurs because they are changing what they are doing. Encourage them to persevere with the techniques, as people usually find that their symptoms gradually decrease, and they are able to do the activities with less discomfort and then increase what they are doing.

- Sometimes people want to do too much – usually on 'good' days when they are feeling better. It is important at these times to encourage them to stick to their programme, as doing too much and not taking planned rests can lead to an unacceptable level of increased symptoms, delay progress and lead to a setback.

- If the person wants you to be actively involved in their programme, it may be helpful for you both to set aside a regular time each week in which to discuss how they are getting on. This will give you the opportunity to reinforce their achievements, give encouragement when they are having difficulties, and discuss any worries that you have in relation to their programme. It is important that you approach any concerns about their programme, whether you think they are doing too much or too little, in a non-judgemental manner.

- Setbacks can occur. They are a 'blip' in the recovery phase and certainly do not mean that the strategies described in this book are not helpful. Setbacks are more likely to occur in certain situations, for example, if the person has another illness, or is going through a busier or more stressful time. These situations may give rise to increased symptoms and an inability to maintain their programme. At these times, it is important to remind the person that setbacks are only temporary. Encourage them to read the appropriate sections of this book to help them to get back on track again. Setbacks should be viewed as challenges to be overcome and not as disasters. If a setback occurs after the person has finished working through the book, then discuss ways to help them get back on track, such as devising a small activity and rest programme for a few weeks, or until they feel they are managing better.

- We hope that, after working through this book, people will feel less fatigued, be able to do more and need less rest. It is important to encourage them to continue with a balance between different kinds of activities and rest. Breaking this routine, or stopping certain activities, or resting at irregular times may lead to a risk of sliding back. As long as a good balance of activity and rest is maintained, recovery is likely to be sustained. They may gradually make quite substantial changes to their lives e.g. returning to work, starting college, or taking over household responsibilities. Although these are all signs of good progress, making these changes can be quite challenging, particularly if the person has been ill for some time. Your support and understanding will almost certainly be appreciated.

Appendix: Seeking professional help outside the UK

Association for Behavioral and Cognitive Therapies in the USA

Website: http://www.abct.org

Australian Association for Cognitive and Behavior Therapy (Western Australia)

Website: https://www.aacbt.org.au/

The European Association for Behavioural and Cognitive Therapies

Website: www.eabct.eu

Index

Note: page numbers in **bold** refer to diagrams.